"Partners 4 Life certainly is a work of passion and love in concert with his donor in trying to make a difference and will touch many lives."

—Susan Stuart,
president and CEO, Center for Organ Recovery and Education;
president, Association of Organ Procurement Organizations

"We highly encourage you and your loved ones read *Partners 4 Life.* Jim Uhrig has diligently researched and chronicled his path before and after IPF (Idiopathic Pulmonary Fibrosis). This is a great resource for those facing IPF."

—Kathleen O Lindell, PhD, RN,
research assistant professor of Medicine
Clinical Nurse Specialist, Simmons Center;
and **Kevin F. Gibson,** MD, professor of medicine
and medical director, Simmons Center

PARTNERS
4 LIFE

Importance of Partners in Surviving an Organ Transplant

Jim Uhrig

iUniverse LLC
Bloomington

PARTNERS 4 LIFE
IMPORTANCE OF PARTNERS IN SURVIVING AN ORGAN TRANSPLANT

iUniverse books may be ordered through booksellers or by contacting:

iUniverse LLC
1663 Liberty Drive
Bloomington, IN 47403
www.iuniverse.com
1-800-Authors (1-800-288-4677)

ISBN: 978-1-4917-2853-6 (sc)
ISBN: 978-1-4917-2855-0 (hc)
ISBN: 978-1-4917-2854-3 (e)

Library of Congress Control Number: 2014904828

Printed in the United States of America.

iUniverse rev. date: 03/24/2014

Partners 4 Life is dedicated to my wife, Donna, who was my personal caregiver. Her role is discussed in great detail in chapter 8, "Caregivers." No words can express my respect for how she handled the stress she experienced during this most difficult time. Dealing with my lung illness, transplant, and the great challenges of trying to survive a double lung transplant while also thriving—these are my daily goals. All caregivers in my family should be acknowledged; I also thank them for their support of me, the patient, and for their excellent support of Donna. On top of managing this health matter, she also maintained our two family businesses—with the help of employees, coworkers, friends, and customers, who might not realize how great their shared expression and compassion meant to Donna.

Caregivers for any transplant patient should earn special wings for their service, and this book is dedicated to all the caregivers and donors for those patients. My donor is the most special partner for life for me. Her oldest son will share the sorrow from the donor side of a transplant, along with those challenges facing the patient and caregivers. *Passion* is one word used by her son—and by many others—to describe her, and ironically this is my demeanor as well. The combined passion from his mother's lungs in my every breath may inspire others to be donors or may help some through the challenge of facing a decision about an organ transplant.

Contents

Without donors there would be no transplants. A potential lung recipient may be focused on his or her next breath, but there would be no more breaths without donors.

Foreword

Accept the Challenges...So that You May Feel the Exhilaration of Victory
—George S. Patton, General, US Army

Very few things in life are more terrifying then the concept of undergoing surgery for an imminently life threatening and otherwise incurable medical problem. Even fewer things in life require the degree of courage that it takes to inhale the anesthetic gas that will render you unconscious and place your very existence squarely in the hands of another person. Almost nothing in life prepares one for the challenge associated with the limitless uncertainty that goes hand-in-hand with having a vital organ replaced with that of another human being. As a cardiothoracic surgeon at a very busy medical center, I have had the opportunity to see many extremely courageous people accept these challenges with the hope of experiencing the exhilaration of renewed health. Jim Uhrig, the author of the book you are about to read entitled Partners 4 Life, is one of those people. As a member of a relatively small group of incredibly courageous individuals who have blazed the path of lung transplantation, Jim has experienced the varied emotions and myriad challenges associate with it and has emerged with renewed life and hope. His story is heartwarming and one that we all can benefit from exposing ourselves to reading. In particular, it is a "must read" for anyone who has had a lung transplant, is trying to decide whether to have one, or is on the waiting list with plans of having one.

Jim's path, like many other transplant recipients, has been marked by frequent and substantial challenge. Many of these challenges are poignantly described in the pages of this book and tell the often untold story of the spectrum of emotion—from faith and confidence to doubt and skepticism—experienced by many patients who have traveled this path. Jim's story is unique, however, in that he has truly taken notice of the very special relationships that are developed between a transplant recipient and the many individuals with whom they cross paths. These "Partners", as Jim aptly call them, are as vital and important as the new lungs sitting within his chest or the immune suppressing medications that protect them. Through the pages in this book, you are transported to an alternate existence in which you can experience the heart sinking disappointment of debilitating illness, the often agonizing physical and emotional challenges of organ transplantation and the absolutely overwhelming exhilaration of renewed life and hope.

The ultimate "partner for life" in transplantation is one that often goes overlooked amidst the hope and excitement of having a transplant— the donor. The generosity and beneficence displayed by organ donors is truly awe inspiring and the number of lives saved due this altruism is staggering. It is certainly the ultimate act of giving without which transplantation would be impossible and survival, for individuals like Jim, unattainable. In his book, Jim describes his experience both with the initial uncertainty and mystery surrounding his donor and ultimately the unique "partnership" he developed with his donor's son that has allowed his donor's story to be shared from her family's standpoint. Just like the life-long partnership Jim will have with his donor, the unique partnerships that he has developed with the many people who have touched his life over the course of his illness and treatment are truly life long and the title of the book certainly embodies that sentiment.

It has been a great privilege to be Jim's lung transplant surgeon and while it has been many years since Jim's operation, I know our unique relationship makes us—Partners 4 Life!

Jay K. Bhama, MD
Cardiothoracic Surgeon
University of Pittsburgh Medical Center

Acknowledgments

Special thanks to Dr. Kathy Lindell of the Simmons Center, Susan Stuart of CORE, Shelley Zomak, and Dr. Jay Bhama for their help and continuous suggestions for *Partners 4 Life*, for they all are just that for me—as are all the personnel at Simmons and nurses and medical support personnel of UPMC. I thank John Sullivan (a former lung transplant recipient) for his mentoring of my illness, getting me ready for the challenge of a lung transplant, and then telling me every day after the transplant, "This is tough, but we will get through it." Then he would pray with my family and me.

Travis Murphy, the oldest son of my donor, friended me through a Facebook search of the US Transplant Games and the members of Team Pittsburgh in those games for 2010 and 2012. That connection and the impetus on his part, has put in perspective the gift of his mother's lungs to me due to her wishes to be an organ donor. She had impact on so many who knew her, and through this book many more will know the spirit in me that I call "Hey Jude."

Extra thanks to my son, Keith, who reviewed portions of the text to add his perspective, particularly in chapter 8, "Caregivers," which is based on his entries in the gratitude journal he started with my wife, Donna.

Lastly, the cover artwork came from Mary Stark, an artist who is the wife of a teammate of mine from Team Pittsburgh. The hat is my signature image, as I wear it constantly for UV protection from the sun; I also like it for the warmth it gives me, since my body temperature is suppressed from the antirejection drugs I take.

Introduction

Partners 4 Life is about the partners I had in my life—and those who came into my life—when I found out I had an incurable disease, pulmonary fibrosis, and would need a lung transplant to survive.

Early in 2008, doing ordinary things literally started to take my breath away. Mundane tasks, like tying my shoes, caused difficulty breathing, and I could not catch my breath. Walking up steps required a stop to rest along the way. Walking up any grade or small hill caused lightheadedness. The natural assumption might be that an overweight male in his midsixties was facing aging issues.

When you have the flu, you normally feel achy, and that is the feeling I had for almost two years prior to my diagnosis. The "good fortune" of catching a bad cold in April 2008 sent me to my primary care doctor. Dr. Mally had been my doctor for close to twenty years, and his casual bedside manner did not alarm me to the serious problem developing in my lungs. Believing I had a bad cold or flu, but not knowing the truth, I wondered why I felt achy all the time and why my strained breathing and shortness of breath was getting worse. Exercise did not help, as it was too exhausting.

When Dr. Mally listened to my lungs, he told me they sounded brittle, like Velcro being pulled apart. He suggested a visit to a pulmonologist and to get chest x-rays and a CAT (computerized axial tomography) scan. That visit and a review of those tests led to a diagnosis of pulmonary fibrosis (PF).

PF was unknown to me, so on my way home that day I made two phone calls. The first was to my wife, Donna, who searched the Internet and found hundreds of pages to print, giving some insight into the disease and treatment options.

The second call was to my friend of forty years, John Sullivan (Sully), who had a double lung transplant in 1997. (See his amazing story in chapter 5, "Sully.") He became one of my most significant and trusted sources in my *Partners 4 Life* saga, as I faced the unknown challenges coming my way.

Sully connected me with the Dorothy and Richard Simmons Center for Interstitial Lung Disease at the University of Pittsburgh Medical Center (UPMC) in Pennsylvania. The Simmons Center—with its staff of professionals dedicated to the research and treatment of pulmonary fibrosis—provided me with an immediate high level of confidence.

Kathy Lindell was my initial contact and was instrumental in my prognosis and getting to the right doctors. She takes interest in every patient, knows how to assess symptoms quickly, and suggests the treatments and adjustments needed to manage a disease that can move quickly.

Dr. Lindell and so many others at Simmons are great partners for life, and she would respond at all hours of the night and day to any question or request.

My lifelong partner and wife, Donna, is very good with medical issues, and our daughter, Robin, is a nurse. When I went to Simmons for my first visit with the medical director, Donna was with me.

The role of caregiver is very important in anyone's illness, but with PF, it is extremely important. Donna could not have done her job better, and when the time came, she had plenty of help from the large family we were blessed with in our lives.

Simmons helped me understand the clinical course of this disease, gave me confidence in treatment options, and reassured me that none of my children or grandchildren had the same fate. That was the single most-driving force in my quest for treatment.

Some self-preservation issues are obvious, but understand what I felt from the beginning: I had been living a full, robust life and had been doing so many things. I never looked back with regrets. There was considerable good luck in my life as well as some close brushes with death; I felt fortunate to gain knowledge about what would likely lead to my demise if untreated. I also felt I had found the doctors who knew the most about this relatively newly identified disease.

I learned from my first visit with Simmons that pulmonary fibrosis had no known cure and that the only solution was a transplant. Patients with this disease faced a limited life expectancy, ranging from a few years to double digits, although that was rare. The clinical course is unpredictable, and a deteriorating condition could decline gradually or in steps. But, in the end, you hit the floor gasping desperately for oxygen.

At the time of my diagnosis in 2008, the medical community did not believe in a genetic link, but from talking to other PF patients, I felt there could be a genetic tendency. My dear mother died of emphysema, which leads me to think that she could have also had PF, as she had similar symptoms. Emphysema and asthma can be misdiagnosed and could be PF. Also, our oldest son, Keith, spent one Christmas in the hospital with a bad case of asthmatic bronchitis.

The latest research indicates a genetic tendency *does* exist, so helping with diagnosis and treatment considerations of future PF patients is a driving force for me. I continue to hope otherwise, but if my family shows tendencies, the Simmons Center can quickly help plan a course of treatment if needed. Scientists have been searching for a cure for a dozen years, and I hope that cure is coming close to a reality, which might eliminate the need for lung transplantation in future PF patients.

Oxygen is critical to the care and treatment of PF patients. Dr. Kevin Gibson, medical director at Simmons Center, did a great job explaining that. After he diagnosed me in May 2008, he started me on oxygen in July after asking, "Do you have any problem carrying an oxygen tank?"

Trying to be a good patient—because listening to the doctor is essential to any chronically ill patient—I told him I would carry oxygen and use it if he felt it was needed. Physical therapy started shortly thereafter. Having professional physical therapists monitoring my oxygen level and heart rate was important for my well-being and strength development.

Dr. Gibson mentioned that lung deterioration, while unpredictable, would progress. By that September, I was touting a bigger oxygen tank, one that could be carried at my side or strapped on like a backpack.

Prescribed oxygen is very important for a PF patient to survive. Without enough oxygen, you can subject your heart to stress, which can lead to pulmonary hypertension—and that can be deadly.

Donna once asked Dr. Gibson about my use of oxygen and suggested that maybe I was using too much and becoming addicted. Dr. Gibson is a great research doctor, and he has a wonderful bedside manner. His response was classic. He smiled and told her, "We are all addicted to oxygen; we cannot get too much."

Oxygen is what we need for life, and PF creates a stranglehold on the air getting to the alveoli sacs in your lungs by hardening the bronchial tubes that provide the passageway to those alveoli sacs. You need more oxygen pushed into your lungs to stop the achy feeling and eliminate that "empty gasping for air feeling" that PF patients can experience.

July 2008 is also when I had a lung biopsy. I was anxious to learn the results while making plans to attend my forty-fifth high school reunion the following week. The lung biopsy is a standard procedure for PF patients, and it required my first stay in the hospital since my senior year of college when I had suffered a football injury.

The biopsy confirmed pulmonary fibrosis, and it confirmed it as idiopathic or a result of an unknown cause, hence the diagnosis of idiopathic pulmonary fibrosis, or IPF.

In my case, I was using oxygen about 50 percent of the time in September, but by Thanksgiving I was on it 24-7, 100 percent of the time. I also steadily increased the levels of oxygen required, all within six months after being diagnosed. I was addicted for sure, but I had access to two large oxygen tank reservoirs and added an oxygen generator for my home office, so it was abundant.

I continued working in my sales job and seeing customers, but I could not go near open flames or high temperature heat sources with my oxygen. I was still traveling to see customers and friends, and I even worked in our family picture framing business during the Christmas rush.

Evaluation for my potential transplant came in early March 2009; it's a very thorough procedure that takes a week in the hospital to complete. All kinds of physical and mental tests are used to evaluate patients for their suitability and possibility of transplant.

I remember well the call from Paul, the pre-transplant coordinator assigned to my case. It came on March 20, 2009; Paul told me I was approved for a double lung transplant and asked if I was sure I wanted to proceed. Without hesitation, I said I was ready, as I knew my oxygen needs were getting more critical, even though I had no idea how bad my lungs were. Besides, Sully had had a lung transplant and was living a full life, so I had a great role model and personal confidence that it could be done.

Within a month, I was blessed with a donor, albeit a high-risk one, because of the donor's age. But it was a donor who my doctors believed was a good match for me. So I had my double lung transplant on April 21, 2009.

That's when fate and luck crushed the family of my donor, Judy, but gave me and my family hope.

An excellent surgeon, Dr. Jay Bhama, removed my old lungs that he later described as "bricks." He estimated that they might have held out another six to eight weeks. Was this timing lucky? Maybe, but the more I learned about my donor, the more blessed I felt. (Her chapter will give you her background and share the agony of a family faced with the sudden loss of its mother.)

After a few setbacks, I came home from the hospital after a two-month stay. I came home without oxygen and was back to work full-time that fall. I also returned to work part-time in our family's custom picture frame business.

The fate of a generous donor gave me new lungs, which came just in time, but my confidence in the medical staff, their competence, and strong support of my wife, family, and Sully, was incredible. All were partners for life and could never be more important than in a transplant scenario.

Having a positive attitude is important, but it sure helps to have supporters rooting you on to keep trying to do your best. My family—especially Donna—and Sully were the best support anyone could ever wish for. But there were so many others who came back into my life to cheer me on with their encouragement of cards, messages, words, and visits, and I will explain some of them in the chapters that follow.

The networking was incredible and culminated in a fundraiser in the fall of 2009 with a golf course full of supporters and diners who helped me raise money for the medication needed until I returned to work. Yes, you can return to work after a double lung transplant. In fact, I still work, with no plans to stop.

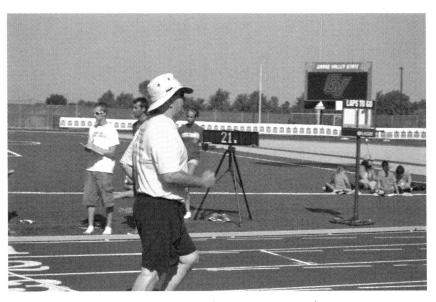

Finishing the 100m race in the 2012 US Transplant Games.

I participated in the 2010 and 2012 Transplant Games, and am planning for the next games in 2014. In 2010, it was as a golfer, and while golf remained some of my focus, I added the one-hundred-meter sprint at the 2012 games. Participating in the games is exhilarating, but having the chance to continue life is a wish any chronically ill person dreams about. Ironically, it is the participation in the Transplant Games that motivated my donor family to seek me out. I had written them of my continuing activity, my plans to write a book, and my desire to get stronger so I could take good care of the gift of their mother's lungs.

The meeting of so many donor families at the Transplant Games is a lasting reminder of the generosity from the gift of life, these people who, through their loved ones, gave me and other transplant recipients a second chance at life. Without donors, most of the recipients would probably not be here, and nor would my many new partners for life and fellow transplant recipients. I wear a *Donate Life* button every day for them and out of respect to the families of donors.

Partners 4 Life gives perspective, and a review of the table of contents will help you follow the story. The importance of partners in my life was natural for me, and before becoming sick it was a way of life for me. From business to sports to just about anything, I always had the good fortune of having great partners who were sought—or somehow they found me. Significant partners are discussed in chapter 4, "Angels," and throughout the book, as they come along often when you need them most, to boost your spirits and give you hope.

If you face a difficult medical problem, stay positive, get the best medical and emotional support, and, if needed, hope for the second chance at life that an organ transplant can give. Work on your physical therapy to rebuild or maintain your strength. Do this under the watchful eye of a trained physical therapist with knowledge of the oxygen needs of a patient with PF. The stronger you can make yourself, the better you will come through the surgery.

Once you are diagnosed, keep learning and listening to those who provide support. Their experience and ideas for your well-being will help you deal with the reality of your plight, and they will help you recognize the options that can lead to your return to a productive life—or perhaps even to a cure for those similarly afflicted.

A return to good health can be inspirational to others who also have the misfortune of developing PF. The disease is a game-changer, but it can be an incredible experience that puts life, family, activities, and life's work in perspective.

There is no time for pity or sorrow... only time to listen to your doctors and your supporters and to get yourself prepared for the challenge of transplant.

CHAPTER 1

Great Partners

Facing the challenge of a possible lung transplant will immediately grab your attention, as breathing is essential to life itself. There is an incredible emptiness and fear when you cannot get air and you gasp for the next breath.

Perhaps someone can deal with this problem alone, but it would be like trying to play golf or tennis alone in a partners or doubles event, never having an extra set of eyes to help find the ball. Paddling a canoe in dangerous waters, or living in the wilderness with no help for survival are other examples; it would help to have a partner to help gather wood, secure food, or just be there for companionship.

There have been many great partners in my life, other than medical ones who came along when they were needed most. The obvious ones during my time of need after my transplant surgery would be my wife, Donna, and my family members. A parent could be a great partner as well. When that partner is a parent and is suddenly lost, as was the case of my donor, the partner for her children and husband is suddenly gone. That person ends up being essential, however, for the person needing a lung or other organ to survive.

Writing this chapter and much of this book, I am at the water's edge of a great western Pennsylvania waterway, French Creek.

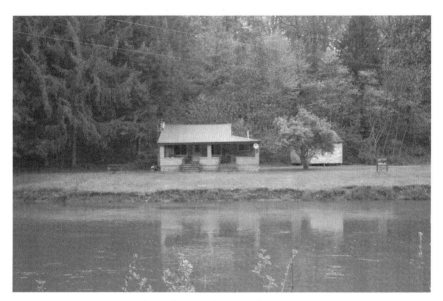

The cabin in the woods, CITW.

The pictures throughout the book, highlighting some of the visualizations, are an attempt to describe the scene better. French Creek is one of the most biologically pure streams in North America, supposedly due to the unique aquatic life present in this river. It flows south from western New York State through the towns of Meadville and Franklin, Pennsylvania. In Franklin, the waters from French Creek flow into the Allegheny River toward Pittsburgh. The Allegheny River is much larger than French Creek; French Creek is normally as wide as a four-lane highway and several feet deep, except for the deep fishing holes along the way.

This chapter is written from the banks of French Creek in a rustic cabin near the little town of Utica, Pennsylvania. Besides the biological uniqueness of this waterway, it has great recreational options for canoeists and kayakers. Canoeing is how I got to learn more about French Creek, through a great partner by the name of Don King.

Don worked for forty years in the same company I did, but he was a generation older. His unique background was that he worked in virtually every department of our company, Harbison Walker Refractories. Refractories are high temperature resistant materials, used to contain hostile environments in industry, like molten metals or intense chemical attack—both of which would destroy a steel shell of a furnace intended to contain those environments. Refractories are the barrier, or—in keeping with the theme of this book—the *partner* needed to keep the heat away from the people operating the industrial furnaces.

Don was quite the authority not only on refractory materials, but also on how to get things done in any part of the company. So, for a less experienced person, he was a great ally.

He went to Allegheny College, on the banks of French Creek in Meadville, PA, as a premed student before serving in the US military in World War II. His college training made him the perfect candidate for being a medic. He served in the European theater, specifically as a medic in the Battle of the Bulge. Don confided in me that the battle provided enough doctoring to last him a lifetime, and instead of going on to med school as his father had, he started his career with Harbison Walker when he returned from the military. With his military medical experience, he would have been fascinated with the technology of organ transplants.

Don had a fifteen-foot, Grumman aluminum canoe that he used regularly on French Creek and other waterways. His son and daughter often accompanied him, but as the years went by, he would often go by himself, paddling his canoe and camping alongside the river.

While enjoying an adult beverage one night after work, Don invited me to join him for an overnight trip on French Creek from the Saegertown access way, about ten miles north of Meadville. Don was about double my thirtysomething age at the time, but he had a zest for life, the outdoors, and nature, and he was a natural tutor and mentor for many.

At that time in his career at Harbison Walker, he was also the advertising manager. I worked closely with him on many publications, technical meetings, and presentations. Don was a great writer with great communication skills; he even taught classes at a local community college in Pittsburgh.

His demeanor was inquisitive; he was always asking questions about how things work, or why do you have that opinion—ever mindful of broadening his knowledge rather than challenging your position. I quickly began to look forward to our canoeing adventures and enlisted other Harbison Walker employees, both young and old, to join us. We often would have two or three canoes for our trips and spend two nights on the river camping in our unorganized "Outward Bound" type program.

Normally, I took responsibility for food and beverages, perhaps because of my sales and marketing background. It more likely resulted from the first overnight trip I made with Don. We ended up sharing a small can of Vienna sausages and one six-pack of beer. Since that trip, Don agreed—perhaps cunningly—to relinquish that duty.

Our relationship grew. After he retired, his wife died suddenly; he sold his house and moved into the apartment in the lower level of our house, south of Pittsburgh. He lived there a couple of years and became part of our family before he moved north to be closer to the water he loved.

When you are in a canoe, you need a good partner. The person in the front helps supply the power, but the person in the back adds additional power and —most importantly—steers. Don almost always sat in the back of a canoe. As he was now into his early seventies, it became more important for my younger eyes to "read" the current and avoid the rocks and submerged objects that Don affectionately called *widow makers.*

There certainly are dangers in the streams and rivers, and many a widow has been made as a result of carelessness or bad luck. One time, on another stream that flows into the Allegheny near Warren, PA we both came close to meeting our fate on a stream called the Brokenstraw. One Saturday afternoon in the spring, we started near Corry, paddled awhile, and then camped near a small island in a steady rain.

At daybreak, that small island was totally submerged and we opted to ride the raging river down to the Allegheny. We made it, but not before dodging many widow makers. More than once, I questioned my judgment, as Donna was pregnant with our son Brad at the time. This was in May of 1982 and Brad was born in August.

A few years later, when our canoe club had six members, we all capsized in the Owassi Rapids on Pine Creek, which flows through the Grand Canyon of Pennsylvania near Wellsboro. As usual, Don and I were riding together. After capsizing, we were able to pull ourselves ashore in a very strong current at the house where Teddy Roosevelt used to fish for trout. As we entered those rapids, there was another canoeing group of Mennonite Boy Scouts from Lancaster, Pennsylvania that were not so fortunate. One of the young leaders died before his twentieth birthday in the near freezing spring waters that day.

Our entire party was visibly shaken by the events and the 38° water. My boss at the time was a gentleman by the name of Dale, and the only thing that saved his life after being in the water for thirty minutes was a raft full of doctors and nurses from Michigan. I alerted them of the incident while they were floating down river and I was running down a railroad right of way—hollering my concern for missing people from both canoeing parties.

They just happened to be coming down river when I yelled brief details to them. They proceeded downstream in earnest and came across Dale, shivering in the water with evident hypothermia. After they picked up Dale in their raft, they brought him to a riverbank where some campers happened to be located. The nurses stripped Dale's clothing from him and then jumped into two sleeping bags with him, to help raise his body temperature.

We laughed nervously about it later, but we all knew it could have been a multiple fatality day on Pine Creek. Dale was an Ohio State grad and big football fan; the nurses were from Michigan, so we told him it was a good thing we hadn't told them he was from OSU, as they would likely not have been so friendly—or such accommodating "partners."

Dale was a great partner for me. He taught me a lot about managing people by working with them, rather than acting as the *boss*.

In my forty-five years in the refractory industry, there were many successes as well as plenty of learning experiences that were *not* successes. But I always tried to take the attitude of a very successful football coach, to blame myself for the losses and give credit to the team for successes. *Partners 4 Life* often can be a team effort, such as with medical teams, family caregiver teams, support groups, each helping others face the challenges of a transplant.

Dale was such a good and knowledgeable boss. He encouraged me to have plenty of outside activities, such as golf, football officiating, and—ironically—canoeing. I was a football official for nearly three decades, working football games in and near the Western Pennsylvania area in both high school and college and later great classic Ivy League college games in the Northeast.

Having had so many great partners from officiating, I could not possibly acknowledge them all, but as I sit on the banks of French Creek, I remember after one game at Allegheny College, my football officiating crew dropped me off at Saegertown access way to meet my friend Don King. What a great memory that is for me, and the officiating crew never forgot it.

For a football officiating crew, the members have to be great partners to be successful, and with my regular crew we had that. Those friendships last a lifetime, and guys like Tic, Woody, Kelly, Linkster, Howdy, Dink, and Charlie were a big part of my success, leading me to work in the Ivy League and many Eastern college games. Often when watching a major college or NFL game, I recognize one or two of the officials, and many I officiated with could have done so.

There are many personal friends who became great partners and really gave me encouragement and support. Many helped give me the courage to face the challenges and hurdles of a double lung transplant. We will review a few in chapter 4, "Angels."

I had many customers who were great partners. The first one who comes to mind is a gentleman called Big Jim who lived in upstate New York. When I was a young sales trainee, one of the first customers who called on the phone was Big Jim. He called asking for some information about one of our products and treated me with the courtesy and respect of a seasoned veteran, rather than a trainee.

Probably ten years or longer went by before I visited Big Jim and also met his three sons, Max, Billy, and Ken. I was sure that Big Jim could not have remembered that telephone inquiry from years ago, but I told him it taught me a lot about dealing with people—that regardless of their experience or background, it was important to treat them with respect.

As I gained experience, I eventually became the regional manager responsible for their business. Through the efforts of a great salesman, Phil, we developed a partnership that grew into the biggest contractor account our company had. It was because they were not just a contractor buying our product; they also allowed Phil to develop a partnership with them selling our products to their customers.

A few years later, my boss, Dale, asked me to run the program for our entire company focused on sales to contractors. It was a tough job and very time consuming, but Dale also allowed me to work with the brightest and best people anyone could hope to have. Stush, DJ, Jerry, Cario, the Petes, and so many others made me look good and we all made it fun and very successful!

I loved that job because of the customers, and I nurtured so many relationships based on partnerships, starting with the signature handshake of the entire program. I could talk about so many of the great relationships of these individual companies. Many of the individuals in those companies were the first to call or write when they heard of my transplant. Many called and talked to my wife, Donna, and gave her such great support that she will never forget it.

One called me a year or so ago. His name was Ted, and he was the son-in-law of the owner of a contractor company. Ted was special. We learned a lot together and played a lot of golf, but also worked all kinds of hours servicing our mutual customers. I told him the remarkable story in this book, and he was amazed how our lives had changed, but that we both had managed to keep the passion of our youthful years.

So many more contractors could add to these stories from coast to coast and especially in the heartland of America, Kansas. This is where my donor came from; ironically, one of the sons of a heartland refractory contractor is involved in transplants there. He works for the Midwestern Transplant Center based in Kansas City, the organ procurement organization that started the process of finding a recipient for my donor's organs.

It is hard to put a value on the partners in our lives, or tell you how great it is to have such partners—whether they were from business, football officiating, personal friends, or, of course, family.

My message to you is that as a patient, you can be uplifted by the people who try to help you get better. If you are a caregiver, a friend of a caregiver, or a friend of the patient, the value of a card, a phone call, a text message, an e-mail, or a personal visit (when allowed) cannot be understated. I had so many supporters, as did my caregivers. I had very little time to think about anything except how blessed I was, bringing me to tears many times, especially when I was starting to take the new powerful drugs needed for my survival after the transplant.

Sully had his caregiver wife, Claudia and our special mutual friend, and his boss, Tom. I never understood why Tom went to see Sully so much, but now I do. He was a busy executive in our company, and he just put such a value on supporting Sully with visits and updates for others to pray for Sully. Thanks to Tom for getting Sully through his ordeals, for I likely would not be here without Sully.

I saved the most important partner for life for last, of course, and that is my benevolent donor. My gratitude for donors is never far from my mind.

Without the gift of her lungs, I would not be looking at this peaceful stream as daylight comes to a close. Her son tells me of her family, who will always miss her dearly, and that she was an advocate of organ donation. Having been an RN, she was familiar with transplant issues. I had corresponded with the family, and they had chosen to be anonymous—which I respected and honored—but in the summer of 2013, four years after my transplant, through the initiative of the oldest son, Travis, a new partner for life was realized. The chapter he wrote about his mother may be one you wish to jump ahead to and read, for while I was adjusting to learning about my new disease, Judy Murphy was helping others as a nurse and training nurses to be aware of organ donorship and transplant issues. Her passion for this helped comfort the family with the delays of the recovery of her organs.

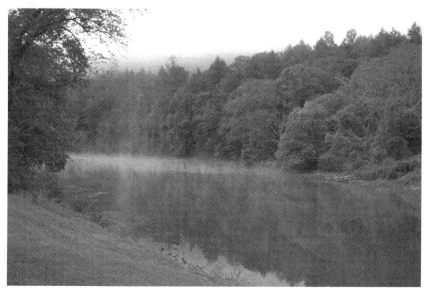

The morning mist coming from French Creek.

Some day, when my work is done and I can no longer watch the peaceful rivers flow, perhaps I will have the honor of embracing my donor and thanking her for the breath of life she has given me, that I have hopefully shared with you.

If you are a patient, this may give you hope.

If you are a caregiver, this may give you humility.

The caregiver role is the toughest part of this whole process. Despite all the good fortune of a timely donor and the marvels of medical expertise, the tears and the stress on the caregiver and donor family are challenging—and perhaps never ending.

I encourage all involved to keep the faith, as God will be with you every step of the way.

Here is part of the eulogy delivered by Travis Murphy, the oldest son, in honor of his mother Judy, my donor, on Thursday, April 23, 2009, two days after her lungs were transplanted to me.

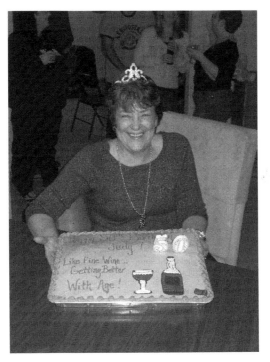

Judy Murphy, *Partner 4 Life*.

Judy Murphy eulogy excerpts delivered by Travis Murphy:

My mom had a keychain for her car keys that read, "I take life with a grain of salt... a wedge of lime, and a shot of tequila."

That was my mom.

It's not until you realize that you will not make any more new memories with someone that you really take a look at the memories you have. And you can more fully appreciate how truly grand they were.

In the midst of everything over the last five days, I have forced myself to pause and remember things about her. Things that I've always taken for granted or that I found annoying that I would now give anything to see her do again.

She had a huge smile and a contagious laugh. It's not until now that I look back at her that I realize how truly happy she always was.

She loved the craziest things.

She loved pigs.

She loved purple.

She loved lilacs and hyacinths.

She loved her family. Like a mother bear. One only had to see her at a high school basketball game in which one of her kids was playing to know that. I don't know that we as her kids appreciated the red-faced woman berating the refs, but you knew whose side she was on.

She loved a story about something interesting. Everything was the funniest, the coolest, the best she'd ever seen or heard. It wasn't necessarily, but to her it was. She would do this thing where she would gasp, and it made you feel like you just told her the most amazing thing. You felt good talking to her. The funny thing was, it was never insincere.

She loved to teach.

She also loved the spring. So it's fitting that we celebrate her life on a day like today. The sun is shining as bright as her smile. She loved the warmth—how could she not, it radiated out from her.

She loved to help people. And she did it throughout her life. And now even in death she does the same. She insisted on being an organ donor. So we as her family and friends can take comfort in that she's still giving, still helping, even in death. Right now, there are families who are now able to spend a few more hours, days, weeks, months with one of their loved ones because of her love of helping others.

We just have to accept the fact that she earned her angel's wings a bit sooner than we would have liked, and her memory and her example lives on as an inspiration to us all.

CHAPTER 2

Medical Partners

Just like the luck of having great partners to get you through normal times in life, when it comes to the partners you need for medical advice, the good fortune of having knowledgeable, well connected partners can help bridge that gap. Hopefully, *Partners 4 Life* will help others think about what to look for in the best medical partner for their health issues. If the patient is suffering from pulmonary fibrosis or another interstitial lung illness, maybe these words will help them the most and connect them with the partners for life they need.

Dr. Mally, my primary care doctor, was my doctor for close to twenty years. I remember walking the halls of his office as he checked my oxygen level with a pulse oximeter. This is done by placing it on your finger, and it indicates your pulse and oxygen level. He also told me when he listened to my lungs that they sounded like Velcro being pulled apart. I later learned that this is typical of pulmonary fibrosis patients; the lungs become brittle, hardening in a way that is indicative of this disease. I was out of breath doing simple things, like tying my shoes, or walking up steps or even a slight grade.

At first, I simply thought I was overweight, out of shape, and just getting older. I never dreamed—nor did my family think—I was as sick as I was. I really think some of the members of my family were not sure of the seriousness of my illness until they saw me in the hospital after my transplant. There was no doubt my condition was severe.

No one hopes to have long lasting medical partners, like a transplant recipient's quest for survival. When diagnosed with pulmonary fibrosis in May of 2008, I had never heard of the disease. The pulmonologist I first visited, referred by my primary care physician, examined me and talked to me about my symptoms. Since he had not told me up to that point what I had, I asked him point-blank, "Do you know what I have?"

Somewhat reluctantly, maybe with bad news in mind, he invited me from the examination room to his office. He showed me x-rays, the CAT scan, and the gray scarring that was apparent in both lungs, but particularly in the right lung. Even my untrained eye could see something was amiss. He then told me, "You have pulmonary fibrosis." He did not tell me much more about the disease and I left with some printed information.

After that first visit to the pulmonologist, my initial reaction was limited by my lack of knowledge of what a diagnosis of pulmonary fibrosis meant. On the way home that day, I made two phone calls. The first was to my wife, Donna, who was at work; having never heard of the disease either, she printed off about a hundred pages of information from the Internet. Later that night, I read every word, twice. Of course, this was after my second phone call made that day, and that was to John Sullivan, who I call Sully.

Sully had a single lung transplant in 1991, and then a double lung transplant in 1997, as the disease that initially destroyed his lungs returned. His disease was called Alpha-1 antitrypsin deficiency, which basically destroys the lungs. He also had a kidney transplant in 2000, because the kidneys are often stressed from some of the drugs needed to treat lung transplant patients. Sully's story is told in chapter 5, "Sully."

I told Sully that the first pulmonologist had said to come back in several months to see how the disease was progressing. He suggested

I get a second opinion, and he placed a call to Dr. Kathy Lindell for my appointment. Thankfully, I listened to my trusted friend and met the medical personnel at Simmons. Instead of waiting for months, I saw the Simmons personnel in a little over a week.

The Dorothy and Richard Simmons Center for Interstitial Lung Disease at the University of Pittsburgh Medical Center was started as a result of a contribution by Richard Simmons to the University of Pittsburgh after his wife, Dorothy, died of IPF in 2001. This center is a research and medical treatment group focused on patients with pulmonary fibrosis and similar lung diseases.

Within a week or so of my initial diagnosis, I was now a patient of the Simmons Center. I began monthly visits to the Simmons Center and was prescribed to start carrying oxygen and to supplement my oxygen level at the beginning of July 2008. If you are a pulmonary fibrosis patient, or have any lung issue that depresses your oxygen level, you need to use the oxygen and level prescribed.

- Oxygen is prescribed for a reason and is a vital medicine for lung issues.
- By not using oxygen you are putting yourself at a large risk, which is unnecessary.

My first contact at the Simmons Center was with Dr. Kathy Lindell, a PhD and RN who had the title of Clinical Nurse Specialist. She was one of the first employees of the Simmons Center, and she is committed to their efforts and the patients they serve—beyond normal expectations. My second contact was my new pulmonologist, Dr. Kevin Gibson, who was the Medical Director for Simmons.

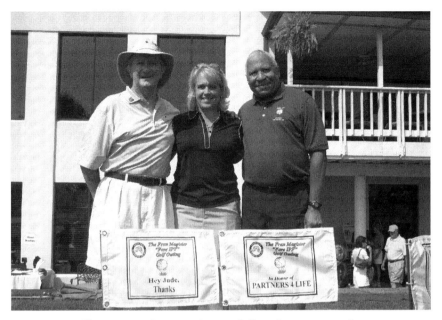

Golf outing with Dr. Kathy Lindell and Dr. Kevin Gibson

From the first visit, I felt a high comfort level with everyone at Simmons—as did my wife—with their knowledge and professionalism. Not only did Dr. Gibson explain things while we were there in his office, but also his penmanship was outstanding and he would write the details of our discussions so you could actually read them.

On that first visit, Dr. Gibson described pulmonary fibrosis as an incurable disease that has a clinical path that goes downward; eventually patients hit bottom because they cannot get enough oxygen. He indicated that the only solution to extend your life would be to get a lung transplant. He put that in perspective by adding that then you have another incurable disease requiring regular medication and exercise, organ rejection can occur, and the new transplanted lungs can fail.

When I asked him for advice on dealing with this disease, Dr. Gibson's response was classic: "Perhaps we should consider to do some travel that we may have been putting off." Not exactly a rosy outlook, but my attitude was that I was getting the best medical care available, and that I had the inside track with Sully as my mentor.

Dr. Gibson really got me moving in the right direction as he gave me my first oxygen prescription in July. Before he gave it to me he asked if I had any reservations about carrying an oxygen tank. I assured him my vanity would not be an issue about such things and that I would do whatever he prescribed.

Simmons is a research facility, so in addition to caring for patients, it has many opportunities for patients to get involved in research studies. However, some patients care not to participate, but my attitude was positive as I felt blessed having such a great life, wife, and family—and I had done things one would never dream of doing. From the beginning, the possibility of there being hereditary issues with my disease also impacted my willingness to face it head-on and not deny it in any way.

Knowing that I had a bloodline of children and grandchildren, I wanted to know about any hereditary issues. I also suspected that my mother, who died when she was well into her eighties, had had similar symptoms—but her death had been attributed to emphysema.

I later learned in my study of pulmonary fibrosis disease that it is often misdiagnosed as emphysema or asthma. This got my attention because of my mother, but also because my oldest son, Keith, had spent one Christmas in the hospital with an asthma attack.

I became a willing participant for any study or examination by the dedicated medical experts at Simmons that they thought could be worthy. Unfortunately, I was not eligible for any of the lung studies, as my body mass index was too high. At least my blood was worthy for those studies.

When I first went on supplemental oxygen in July, I really only used it for exercise. The tank was small, about the size of a football. I remember actually running with it like a football at the local high school field, reflective of my football playing and football officiating days. I figured I was doing pretty well, and carrying a little football-sized tank was not that difficult. Two months later, the tank was twice as big, as a higher level of oxygen was prescribed; I was unsuccessful when trying to run with that size of a portable tank like a backpack.

At home in our long ranch style house, we also went from one large storage tank for oxygen to two large storage tanks for each end of the house. Since I was still working in my sales job and traveling, a little tank was strapped on the backseat of the car so I could travel overnight. On one trip, that little tank needed to be refilled along the way. The Simmons personnel were always on top of any of my needs, no matter where I was or what I was doing.

I called that little backseat tank *R2-D2*, after the droid of the same name in *Star Wars*. I can assure you that when you're relying on an oxygen tank for breathing, you have no visions of being a Jedi, yet I was able to continue to work, right until the day I was called for my transplant in April of 2009, eleven months after being diagnosed.

Roughly six months after being diagnosed, I had two large storage tanks in the house, *R2-D2* in the car, and an oxygen generator in my home office. As my condition worsened, the need for more oxygen was obvious, so I started to avoid overnight travel and any airline travel.

To say that the Simmons personnel were great is an understatement. I became more involved in the patient support group, and Simmons continues to host a support group on a monthly basis. This is still a priority for me because of their concern for all their patients.

I'm one of the lucky ones. While I feel that luck perhaps had something to do with it, I wonder if perhaps I had been blessed for other reasons and that maybe this book will help others similarly challenged. If this book is some help for other patients—or perhaps for medical personnel making progress in finding a solution for this disease—or if it helps aid in the awareness and understanding of this disease, then that is important to me. Hopefully none of my offspring will get this disease, but if they do, there is hope that the medical research experts will find a cure in the near future.

When I was diagnosed with this disease in 2008, we were told there was no cure and it was not hereditary. It was reported in 2012—through independent gene studies by three different research groups—that there *are* genetic tendencies.

Also in 2012, they reported that within the next several years they could have a cure for pulmonary fibrosis and that transplants may not be needed in certain cases. In cases where transplants still may be necessary, there is optimism about research into the stem cell area; new lungs could possibly be developed by the patient's stem cells. If this technology comes to fruition, then the patient would not need the antirejection drugs, such as I take twice a day, religiously.

There are many other medical personnel who were instrumental to me, such as the nurses and staff of the ICU and the transition floor. They were wonderful! When I visit the hospital I make a point to acknowledge everyone I recognize, and I hug the ones whom I gave the most trouble during my stay.

My surgeon, Dr. Jay Bhama, was excellent, and although I often stop by his office to say hello, I rarely find him there because of his busy schedule. Perhaps you will get a little insight into the quality and passion of this transplant surgeon from the foreword he wrote for this book. Not only would he not let me quit when I had some tough times, but also he went out of his way time and again to reassure my family—especially my wife, Donna—that things were going to be okay. Despite how bad I felt, when I saw him standing in my doorway or at my bedside, I agreed with his perspective—things *were* going to be okay.

The last person to acknowledge in this section is Shelley Zomak. Shelley is the Unit Director RN responsible for cardiothoracic transplant patients from the time they get the call to after they get out of the hospital and have questions or need follow-up. I met Shelley for the first time at our frame shop in September of 2008. She had come into our store to have some frames made. I was in the back room framing, and my wife, Donna, waited on Shelley and her mother; the subject was an old wedding picture of her mother and father.

After that transaction was completed, Shelley then pulled out five certificates she was presenting to different entities for the assistance they gave at the US Transplant Games in Pittsburgh in August 2008. Upon seeing the certificates, Donna asked Shelley where she got them and what her role was. Shelley then explained simplistically what her duties were at UPMC for transplants.

At that point, Donna stepped back from the counter and called me to the front room. As I came around the corner carrying my backpack of oxygen and saw Shelley and her mother in our store, I developed even more positive feelings for UPMC and the idea of a transplant. As it turns out Shelley, was the transplant coordinator who had called Sully when he got his double lung transplant in 1997, so again I got an additional dose of confidence knowing I had the best possible medical people looking after me and encouraging me.

In the almost five years since my transplant, I've been back for routine examinations and tests of my new lungs. Lung recipients must realize that success can end and that they may need to go back for some additional medical treatment.

In the meantime, I'm going to do what I told the nurses in ICU. "I want to be a good patient—please tell me what I need to do, and thank you."

CHAPTER 3

Simmons Center

The impact the Simmons Center has had on my life certainly makes it deserving of its own chapter, and it continues to help so many patients. This chapter will tell you more about this wonderful health center dedicated to the care and treatment of interstitial lung disease.

The Dorothy P. and Richard P. Simmons Center for Interstitial Lung Disease was created in 2001 by a generous gift from the Simmons family, after the death of Richard Simmon's wife, Dorothy, to this disease.

The Simmons Center is dedicated to providing the highest quality healthcare, education, and support for pulmonary fibrosis patients, mostly dealing with idiopathic pulmonary fibrosis (IPF), as well as providing support for patients, caregivers, and loved ones. Scientists and physicians at this center engage in leading-edge research, aimed at finding a cure for IPF and other interstitial lung diseases, including sarcoidosis and other types of pulmonary fibrosis.

IPF is the most common form of interstitial lung disease, indicated by progressive scarring of the lungs that gradually interferes with the ability to breathe. The diagnosis of IPF is challenging, maybe frightening, as there are no known proven therapies; lung transplantation remains the only option for longer term survival. IPF places a great burden on patients and their families.

Sarcoidosis is another common interstitial lung disease that affects many people in a variety of ways, most commonly affecting their lungs and their ability to breathe.

Optimal care depends heavily on a team of specialists, whose complimentary skills provide each patient with a full range of options. Through the Simmons Center and its evaluation and treatment by a multidisciplinary team, patients receive the full capabilities of the University of Pittsburgh Medical Center. University of Pittsburgh researchers and clinicians at the Simmons Center also work closely to translate basic research on interstitial lung disease into new medical treatments that hopefully will save lives in the future.

If it were not for my friend John Sullivan directing me to the center, I probably wouldn't have known about it. This was after my first visit to a pulmonologist who diagnosed my disease and set me up for a follow-up appointment a few months later. But after I talked to Sully on my ride home from that pulmonologist, he helped me schedule an appointment at Simmons Center the following week, where I felt an immediate comfort and confidence level from their impressive and knowledgeable expertise.

Because the work of Simmons is primarily dedicated to the disease I had, (IPF), I felt I was getting the best care *and* the opportunity to work with research specialists to help find a cure for this disease. This was really important to me; genetic issues were a possibility, and I have four sons and grandchldren from a bloodline that could have also included my mother.

My mother died in her mideighties from emphysema, but I have since learned that emphysema and asthma are often misdiagnosed, for they could really be pulmonary fibrosis. Her difficulty in breathing and other issues were very similar to what I experienced.

As with me, her lung problems manifested themselves over a short period of time in her later years. With that knowledge—and talking to other IPF patients who had the same suspicions of a genetic link from their parents—I really wanted to know more.

I dealt with a lot of research and problem solving in my education and work background, so I felt right at home with the research-oriented Simmons personnel. When I asked about genetics after I was first diagnosed in 2008, I was told there was no confirming research at that time in support of that concern. More recently, in 2012, Simmons and two other research centers concurrently concluded that there *is* a genetic tendency, which was important news to me.

The concern of my offspring being stricken by this disease will always be there for me, but I'm comforted by the fact that the progress being made by Simmons and other research facilities may lead to a cure for this disease in the future.

When you deal with a research center such as Simmons, you have the opportunity to participate in numerous research studies. I was enthusiastic to participate, but my body mass index did not qualify me for any research other than blood studies. Let me just say I was well over my football playing weight—and even over my football officiating weight.

Regardless of my personal situation, there were plenty of other patients who met the criteria of the studies and who became willing participants. This came from the strong support group hosted by Simmons—of which I have been an active participant since my first meeting in June of 2008.

My wife was not such a willing participant; perhaps she was fearful of the diagnosis or in denial of the severity of the disease and the resulting prognosis leading to my demise. I just wanted to know more, as my bloodline might be involved. I really did not know what my chances were and how they could be impacted, but I was certainly listening intently to my medical partners.

My overall attitude was that I had a great life, a wonderful family, and that I did more fun and meaningful things than I ever dreamed one could possibly do. No way was I shortchanged in any manner, and just maybe I could help my offspring or other patients. If indeed I needed a transplant, I was in the best place possible.

UPMC has now done over three thousand lung transplants, and it routinely does more than any other transplant center in the United States. The combination of the two groups—Simmons, with its specialization in pulmonary fibrosis, and UPMC—increases patients' probability for the best treatment and gives them the best chance for a transplant, if that is what they need.

Simmons Center patients come from all over the world. If you become their patient, you will find them expeditious in their assessment of your condition, and they will give an excellent explanation of the benefits of their treatment ideas and research studies. If you choose to be proactive, you likely will feel better about yourself. This could not only help others, but also maybe make you a prime beneficiary of the work.

Participating in a clinical study has both risks and benefits. Your doctors or those at Simmons Center can explain them best. The Simmons Center studies are well designed and well executed, and they often involve more than one research center, as they are part of a network of multicenter studies across the United States. Their studies may give the patient access to new research treatments, and the patient gets regular and careful medical attention during the study.

Of course, the benefits balance against the risk of side effects, which can be unpleasant, serious, or even life threatening. The study will likely require more of a time commitment than standard treatment would, with all the related additional issues from blood work to dosage treatments. Despite the risks, I was more than willing to participate in whatever way the Simmons personnel suggested.

Having an incurable disease such as idiopathic pulmonary fibrosis—with the only option being a lung transplant—certainly can change your perspective, and for me it was an easy choice. Other than being overweight at the time, I was mentally and physically strong, which ironically made me a better transplant candidate when the time came.

If you have any interstitial lung disease issues, I encourage you to contact the Simmons Center (http://www.upmc.com/services/pulmonology/interstitial-lung-disease/pages/default.aspx) for their assistance and professional advice. There are also two advocacy organizations for patients with pulmonary fibrosis. One is the Coalition for Pulmonary Fibrosis (http://www.coalitionforpf.org) and the other is The Pulmonary Fibrosis Foundation www.pulmonaryfibrosis.org.

Keep the faith.

CHAPTER 4

Angels

Perhaps the most pleasant memories of my transplant dealt with my awareness of the presence of angels. Whether you believe in angels or not, if you experience a serious medical situation like a double lung transplant, you are likely to believe in anything that can give your mind hope. I cannot say that before I started my transplant ordeal that I believed angels existed. I now do believe that angels are messengers from God who help give you comfort and perhaps a better understanding of the situation at hand.

One of the most remarkable occurrences was the presence of angels to help me gather strength and face challenges as my illness got worse. During my hospital stay, many were present, but they started "gathering" long before I even knew I was sick. They came in and out of my life as I think angels sometimes do, but they helped me realize I was not alone, and many would be there for my support if needed. They all gave me warmth and comfort, and some have stayed in my life to help look after me and give me continuing hope.

Many people believe in angels, and while I did not acknowledge them before I got sick, I realized how important they were to me as I became more ill. Perhaps some were sent unknowingly to help me through the challenges I would face. Their wings gave me warmth and lifted my spirit, and their touch reassured me they would be with me. They weren't necessarily with me every moment, but they made their presence felt in many ways.

Some angels were people who helped communicate my condition to the caring network that had assembled and followed my progress. They got most of their information from Sully, who has earned his wings over and over in his attention to transplant patients at UPMC.

Sully is also a Eucharistic minister, so he has access to areas like ICU and other areas normally only available to direct family members. Sully came to see me just about every other day and often every day, and his comments were normally along the lines of *this is tough, but we're going to get through it*, and then he would say the Lord's Prayer with me. His knowledge of lung transplants through his personal experiences helped him communicate the key issues to my family and my principal caregiver, my wife, Donna.

Since I had known Sully for over forty years, we had built a personal rapport and relationship as both friends and business colleagues. When Sully was going through all of his transplant issues, I lost touch with him, and quite honestly, the reports of his demise were common. He got the last rites on more than one occasion, but he fought on and is living a productive life—still working, golfing, and ironically, he outlived his dear wife, who died of cancer a year or so before my transplant.

Sully introduced me to the personnel at the Simmons Center and notably Dr. Kathy Lindell, who wears her angel wings every day. She is so dedicated to the patients that come to the Simmons Center, and she is always responsive to questions or needs no matter the time of day or day of the week. She was my first contact when I contacted Simmons, and I have forwarded many other patients to her whom I felt could be helped by the Simmons personnel. Besides handling all of the medical issues, Kathy serves as the liaison for the Simmons Patient Support Group for patients with interstitial lung issues.

The next significant angel who came into my life was Shelley Zomak. Earlier, I talked about meeting Shelley when she came into our frame shop one Saturday morning in September 2008. I had been diagnosed with IPF a few months earlier and had been carrying a portable oxygen tank since July. In September, when Shelley and her mother showed up at our frame shop, I had the backpack variety for my oxygen needs, which were increasing. Shelley is the unit director of the cardiothoracic transplant personnel, who look after patients who need a transplant—but she also is the coach of Team Pittsburgh for the US Transplant Games.

Shelley came to get something framed, but perhaps her angelic mission was the driving force. There are plenty of other frame shops she could have visited, but what brought her to ours is perhaps a mystery of faith. With her nursing career focused on transplants, she gave me great comfort in knowing someone else who would be important in my transplant journey.

I could go on and list many other angels who are nurses, as there are many. Whenever I visit the hospital, I make a point when I see any of the nurses or medical personnel who were involved in my care to thank them personally and show them my continuing improvement. I try to do special things for them at certain times of the year, and occasionally I send a card for their bulletin boards.

Here is a recap I wrote in 2011 after I visited the cardiothoracic ICU area of UPMC one day and saw Angela, a special nurse there:

Had some routine tests at Falk Clinic and did well on them. I gave a copy of the *Taking Flight* book, filled with inspirational stories of lung transplants, compiled by Joanne Schum, to a technician who is in the PFT (Pulmonary Function Test) area and a friend of Sully's and mine. The technician's name is Joanne also, and she is always supportive and watchful, so I gave her a book and told her all about it. She could not thank me enough. I have learned over the last three years of her giving me PFTs—plus she has been doing Sully's PFTs a lot longer— that she is an angel behind the scenes and deserves a few comments and hugs... angels bring out the best in the hug department!

She has introduced other patients to me in the waiting area of the Falk Clinic area where we all go for tests and to see the docs. She knows I will try to help those patients with my positive attitude. I have exchanged e-mails with many of them and have received appreciative comments.

When I went to ICU, I visited a patient I met from South Carolina through mutual friends, and Angela used me as a poster boy at his door. Maybe I helped, for he had a tough time, but appeared to be doing better and he recognized me.

While I was in ICU, I got to know Angela, who is a special RN, for spirit uplifting. She was very special to me, and especially to Donna, my wife, and used to take me to an outside garden to get some fresh air. You have to understand, I was in ICU for a long time and after the first week, came back for another month, and it wasn't because of the good cookin'!

Angela gave me all the care and nursing one could ever hope for. She would pack me up when I was getting better the second time in ICU, and would take me outside to the garden. The first time she did this she told Donna we were going on a date. It had to take her an hour to get everything lined up to take me outside, with monitors, IVs, and back-ups in a really big wheelchair.

Well, we got to the garden, and I said, "Wow, this is really nice. Now can I go back inside and lie down?" Seriously, I was tired and worn out just getting ready to go outside, as sitting up was a chore for me at times in ICU. She took me out several other times, and I may have even taken a nap once, and one time had dinner.

Angela was special. I found out later she would take some patients there when there was little hope, and some passed there. I guess I figured with all the trouble she went to getting me there, I should not let her down.

She also loved the *Taking Flight* book and had me sign my story. I told her that her task was to get every UPMC patient to sign her book. It was a special day. Angela called me one year (2012) right before Christmas, and what a great chat we had. I need to pay her a visit to tell her about my continuing recovery.

Besides medical angels, I had so many other angels looking after me. The first one was Karen Lee, who came back into my life in January of 2008, long before I knew I was sick. Karen Lee was the head majorette of our high school, and she called to raise my interest in attending our forty-fifth high school reunion. She made an enthusiastic pitch to have me attend the reunion, which I had never done before. Maybe it was her charm, maybe it was her enthusiasm, but I committed to go to that reunion, long before I knew I was sick or how much I knew those old friends would be needed to keep my spirits up.

The next angel came in the form of Mickey, an old college teammate of mine. We played baseball together, and he played basketball in college while I was a football player. Mickey made me aware of a dinner where they would be hosting basketball players in honor of the great basketball tradition of our college.

One of the many jobs I had in college was as the statistician of the basketball team, so Mickey asked me to join him for the dinner. I wasn't going to go, but at the last minute something inspired me to do so, and I spent an evening with people I hadn't seen in over forty years. Now Mickey has never been labeled an angel, but he is a great guy. Like Karen Lee, he put me in touch with many old friends long before I even knew I was sick.

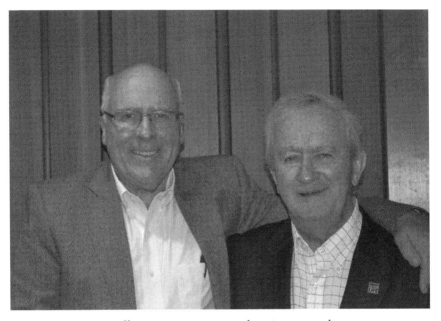

My college roommate, Dr. John Simms, and me
at a Bethany College Celebration

Those friends rallied others around me and encouraged me to fight for my survival. Sully told me it was going to be tough, but we would get through it.

Two other significant angels—two high school friends—came to my aid and support after my transplant. The first was Herk, who walked into ICU on more than one occasion to visit me. I had not seen Herk in forty-five years, other than at that high school reunion, so it took me a minute or two to realize it was Herk and not a long-lost brother as he told the nurses' station. Herk retired from the Air Force after a very successful career. He helped communicate my condition to my other high school friends, and the result was more cards and letters than I could ever imagine.

Quite a few cards were from Barb, a high school friend and cheerleader who kept cheering me on to get better. In high school, I was very close to Barb and her twin brother, Lee, although I had not seen them since high school. Lee died thirty years ago of a heart attack. Even in high school, Barb was a volunteer in the hospital and always had a caring touch for others, as she does to this day. She became a schoolteacher and always had a positive, encouraging nature.

Karen Lee referred to herself and Barb as *Jimmy's Angels* after the television show popular in our youth. They certainly worked some miracles in communicating my condition and helping generate the prayers and thoughts that helped my recovery through some dark periods.

God bless all the angels in my life. They made a tremendous impact on me, and many times while I was looking at their notes and cards in the hospital, I appreciated their presence more than they will ever know. I hope to repay their kindness if the opportunity presents itself.

They are true partners for life, and I encourage anyone facing a similar condition to recognize your partners for life who may be sent unknowingly as angels to lift your spirits and give you hope.

CHAPTER 5

Sully

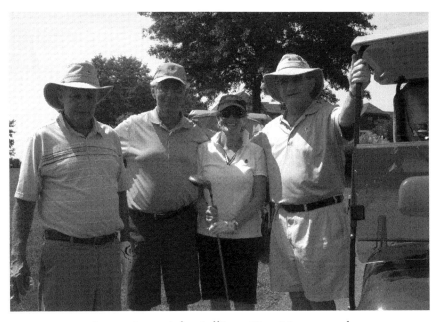

George Geyer, John Sullivan, Vera Maynor, and
me at 2013 Simmons golf outing

John Sullivan is a *"Hall of Fame"* angel to me. He first came into my
life in 1970 when we both worked for a refractory company called
Harbison-Walker based in Pittsburgh. John and I were both young,
new employees trying our best to understand what would be our
chances in working for a medium-sized company. We were both in
the technical marketing area of the company, giving support to our
customers and the salespeople who called on accounts that used these

products. John and his new bride, Claudia, were easy to like, friendly people, and as a coworker he was serious and dedicated to his role.

There were two major markets in the company. One was focused on big steel companies who used the most refractory, and the other was all other industrial type accounts. Refractories are used in high temperature industrial applications to contain the molten metals and gasses up to three thousand degrees and higher.

John worked servicing the steel customers, and I ended up in the industrial market. Over the next twenty years we would see each other occasionally at sales meetings and management meetings as we both progressed to sales management jobs. Here is John's story as told in the book *Taking Flight: Inspirational Stories of Lung Transplantation*. As you see, he was a trailblazer patient in the lung transplantation field. His fighting was not apparent to me; I only knew he was very sick. Not only did I not understand what he went through, but also I had no idea what a role model he would be for me.

John Sullivan's story in his own words:

In 1981, at the age of 35, I (John Sullivan) was diagnosed with Alpha 1 antitrypsin deficiency, which is a genetic disease where your own body tears down your lungs. The doctor told me that I wasn't going to die in 2 years but that I would not live a normal life. At that time I had no idea what he was talking about. My children were 8 and 6 and all I could think about was getting my children through college.

I continued to work and my lungs continued to deteriorate until in 1989 I was on oxygen 24 hours a day. A doctor said that I might want to consider a lung transplant. First of all, I had never heard of a lung transplant, and secondly, I wondered: *how could I be sick enough to even consider one?* In 1990 I was evaluated at the University of Pittsburgh and put on the lung transplant list. At that time they were going to give me a heart and lung; I did not have any idea what to expect because I had never even met anyone that had any type of transplanted organ. I continued to work and after 14 months, April 30, 1991, I got the long anticipated call. I received a single right lung.

I was in the hospital for about 5 weeks and then went home with no oxygen and resumed my life. I did very well for about 6 months until on 11/2/91 I came down with pancreatitis. I was air-lifted from Michigan back to Pittsburgh to be treated. The pancreatitis was caused by the medicine and when the meds were adjusted to cure the pancreatitis, my right lung rejected. I went home after 3 weeks cured but when my body rejected my transplanted lung it reduced my lung capacity by about 50%. I went back to my "normal life." I was huffing and puffing but not back on oxygen.

In April of 1994 I came down with a fungus called *aspergillus.* With the fungus, my lung capacity continued to deteriorate to a point that I would spend the next 3 months in the CTICU trying to get off a respirator and they told my wife 4 times I was not going to make it. As hard as I tried I could not get totally off the machine. I was placed back on the lung transplant list and finally went home to wait, using the respirator at night.

I started to work at home from an office connected to my bedroom. It was very important for me to work because it took my mind off of my illness and the fact that I was waiting for another transplant. I waited for 32 months when in October of 1996 I got the long awaited call. We flew to Pittsburgh and I was wheeled into the operating room and hooked up to all of the lines when the word came down that there was something wrong with the lungs and there would be no operation. Claudia, my wife, and I stayed the night in the hospital and in the morning rented a car and drove back to Detroit to start the wait again.

Once again in Jan 1997 we got the call and flew to Pittsburgh, but when we got to the hospital we were told that the lungs were unable to be retrieved from the donor. I was so sick at that time I was put back on the respirator and went into the CTICU. After a few weeks in the CTICU, I was taken to 7-D to again wait for a suitable set of lungs.

The doctors were concerned with my poor kidney function, as well as my lung capacity, and because of the kidney problem, I was taken off the list, even though I had been on the list for three years. It was Dr. Bartley Griffith who put me back on the list, because he believed in me. On Feb 4, 1997, a suitable set of lungs became available in Augusta, GA. I received the double lung transplant but the operation was too much for my kidneys and I lost them. When I came out of the operation I was in a coma and on dialysis. After 2 weeks I came out of the coma and went to the step down floor to recover my strength. At that time I only weighed 106 pounds and could not sit up, roll over, or walk. After 3 months I went home.

I was on dialysis but that was okay because I could breathe again. I worked very hard trying to regain my strength. I would sit in a lawn chair in my driveway, and could only walk between mailboxes on my street, sit down and rest, and try to do it again. After about 2 months I could walk halfway around the block, and one night my wife and I were walking our dog when a friend came to see us. At the same time the leash got caught on my legs, I bent down to undo the leash when the dog ran off and I fell in the road. I knew at once something was wrong. The ambulance took me to the hospital and I found out that I had broken my left hip. Three pins were put in my hip and after 4 days I was again back home. I was doing ok on my walker when 10 days later, as I was sitting in my chair, I had a grand mal seizure that drove my femur through my pelvis on my right hip and bent the ball over on the previously broken left hip. My doctor did not know if I would ever walk again. He put me in traction for about 6 weeks and then I came home in a wheel chair. A year later I was playing golf with my doctor and complained that I could not get the distance I used to get. He commented that last year he did not know if I would ever walk again. That comment put the golf game in the right light.

I was still on dialysis and in need of a kidney transplant. In 1998, my wife and I decided to move to Pittsburgh so if I were lucky enough to get a kidney transplant it would be at the hospital that knew my lungs. In January 2000 I received a kidney transplant.

Now my kidney is working well and they tell me that my lungs are better than 98% of the people in the world. We had come a long way after 20 years of battles.

As I mentioned, my main goal was to get my children through college. Both of them have graduated and my wife has just finished graduate school. In May of 2000 I also was able to walk my daughter down the aisle. That was very emotional for me because I never thought that I would be here for that special occasion. I now have 3 grandchildren who love their grandpa very much.

I have been to 3 transplant games where I participated in golf and never even thought about winning. I know that I have already won the biggest challenge of my life. I am going to the games to participate in something that would not have been possible without the support of my wife and family, friends, medical staff, and Dr. Griffith who believed in me. Even with all of my support, I know that without the love and generosity of the donors and their families I would not be telling my story today.

Thanks to all of you, I *now have my life back!*

This is quite a remarkable story, and John continues to work and enjoy the grandchildren whom he adores, traveling often to New England to spend time with them. His dear wife, Claudia, developed lymphomatic cancer and died within a year and one half of her being diagnosed. That happened in 2007 and the devastating loss of his caregiver and partner for life was understandably very difficult for him.

His interest in transplant patients and their caregivers keeps him motivated to help on a regular basis at UPMC, specifically with transplant candidates and potential candidates. His Eucharistic minister skills are often called upon, and they give him access to areas like ICU and even the operating areas to check on and give feedback to families—as he did for mine when I received my transplant.

He gave so much comfort to my wife, Donna, and was a supporter as much for her as he was to me.

Guilt and love are often conflicting feelings for the transplant patient. Combined with the caregiver's pain watching all of the suffering, those feelings can make complete recovery of the relationship difficult. As in the case of Claudia, her own demise came as a result of cancer. Often the caregiver's own resistance or health is compromised.

The caregiver needs to get breaks from the stress of the routine with help from friends and family, to stay occupied with something other than worrying about the patient; this is normally difficult for most caregivers.

CHAPTER 6

The Call

The call is the moment the phone rings and you are told that a donor's organs are available. It is a very tense time for recipients and their family and friends. Just imagine what it would be like for you, if you had to get that call. That is a very real scenario to potential organ recipients, as every time the phone rings after activated for a lung transplant, your anticipation escalates.

If you get the call, the next question the pre-transplant coordinator will ask you is whether or not you will accept the organ. In the case of a vital organ like lungs or heart, this can be a very stressful time for the recipients and their families. Thoughts of the donor family likewise will enter into almost everyone's mind, but the focus is on the recipient as soon as the call is received.

Other questions will be about your current health. If you have a fever, cold, or the flu, you will not be acceptable. I have had personal friends who were waiting for a transplant and had organs come available, but because of their high fever the surgeon rejected their candidacy.

There can be other questions, as in my case when my donor was identified as a high-risk donor. The coordinator explained that this was because of age, as my donor was in her early fifties. While I was not aware of the likelihood of another donor, I indicated that I was ready.

If the doctors felt they were worthy to be transplanted, I accepted, and we had to get to the hospital as soon as possible.

The caller also told me that my surgeon would be Dr. Jay Bhama. I had confidence that all of the transplant surgeons at UPMC would be excellent for my surgery, and with the severe condition of my lungs, I had no idea how bad they actually were.

I took a shower, suggested by the coordinator, and was calm and relaxed. I drove my wife and myself to the hospital where we checked in at the emergency room. They were all set for me as they were alerted of the situation by the coordinator. Without breaking any traffic laws or taking risks, we arrived at the hospital a little over an hour after I got the call.

Because I was working right up to the day of the call, before I left home I sent a prepared e-mail to my boss and copied the president of the company:

Subject: The Call Came

I am on my way to Presby.

Donna will call Gus in AM

Peace...............

JRU

I was being prepped for surgery early the morning of April 21, 2009. With five kids and three brothers, we had a lot of people to alert. My wife did an excellent job letting everyone know, and if she was nervous she did not show it to me. (Two months prior to my transplant she had her right shoulder totally replaced, so she always was pretty tough physically and mentally, and she rarely complained.) I was not nervous, thanks to all the preparations by my medical partners and the advice Sully had given me; more importantly, I had an inner feeling of peace.

I would say I am not overly religious, but I have good Christian values and a broad religious background from my youth and college days. I carried a small (one by two-inch) steel cross with me which is inscribed *Jesus Christ is Lord*, given to me by a fellow Rotarian.

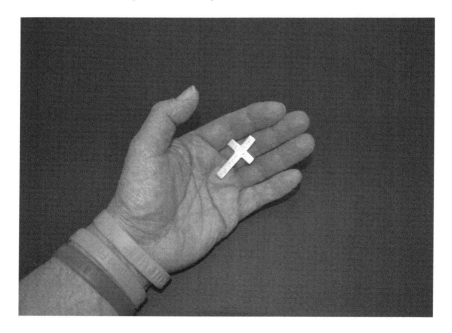

During my surgery and in the early days in ICU, I had to rely on my family to keep track of the cross, but most of the time I was clutching and rubbing the cross with my thumb, as I do every night to this day, even though the cross I had in the hospital has been replaced.

I guess you could say I am a believer in faith, and my signature phrase to others with medical issues, is to *keep the faith*.

I was evaluated for my transplant the first week of March, and on the twentieth of that month, I got the word that I was approved for a double lung transplant. Paul was the coordinator who called me and asked me the same question I received the night of *the call*. His question was simple:

"Are you sure you are committed to go through with the transplant?"

I responded positively.

Paul e-mailed me April 2013—a week before I got the call—and wrote this:

> *LAS increased to 43.6478, a pretty good score. And top of our (UPMC) list.*

The LAS is a Lung Allocation Score and is a rating assigned to the patient indicating the relative need and condition of the patient. The LAS numbers are from 1 to 100. The higher risk and sicker you are, the higher the number. This could be partly due to your lung issues, but it could also be from other issues as well; a lower number would indicate you are not as bad. If your number is too high, the odds of you making it through the surgery decrease, and accordingly this could eliminate you from getting the call.

I was getting close to getting the call, and I was staying cool and collected.

In my case, I had Sully and also had great confidence in the competence of all the medical professionals at UPMC. The Simmons Center personnel and specifically the support group gave me a lot of confidence that others had been through this procedure and done well. Certainly there was a risk, but I also had seen other members of the support group who did not get a transplant and were no longer with us.

The support group meetings help you set the stage for your journey through a simple part of each meeting. At the beginning of each meeting, each participant talked about the status of his or her situation. Those who have received transplants offer their encouragement by their presence and especially by their sense of well-being. Those battling pulmonary fibrosis were in the same situation as I was, and we were all learning from each other as well as from the medical professionals, who were my new partners from the Simmons Center.

With all of the doctor visits, support meetings, talking to other patients in dealing with my disease, and my increasing need for oxygen—it was easy for me to accept the challenge of a lung transplant. Again, my longtime friend, Sully, could not have been a better role model. As you read in his chapter, Sully was not only a great role model, but also he really became a true hero to me. We continue to be great friends, and Sully has helped many lung transplant recipients at UPMC.

If you are considering a lung transplant or any transplant, you need to give serious consideration to how you will react when you get that call. If you are fortunate like me, you may only have to go through it once, but others are not so lucky and never get the call. Others may go to the transplant center and get rejected because of something wrong with the donor lungs. That happens, so you need to be prepared for that possibility, which is very stressful to everyone with your interest at heart. Stay cool and keep the faith.

My surgeon, Dr. Bhama, confided with my family after the surgery that I was the fourth lung transplant he had performed in the last six days, which made him think that, given the odds, something would occur to cancel my destiny with my donor. I thank God that all of the variables connected, but I often rub my cross and think of my donor and her family. I have a sense of closeness with my donor that is comforting and often emotional.

I wish you well in your transplant decision and offer comfort to your family to support you like my family supported me. Should you decide not to get a transplant—or if some unfortunate circumstance prevents the process from going smoothly—my best advice is to keep the faith.

I had confidence, and here is one last example of an e-mail I sent to my sales team, as I was their general sales and marketing manager and felt good about what I was undertaking. Here is what I told them when I got that first call from Paul, the pre-transplant coordinator, telling me I was added to the list:

Subject: First Day Of Spring (2009)

Well tomorrow is the first day of spring and also the first day of my being on the active transplant list.

If I get that call, I will get the word to Gus, who can share this with you all. You all know some of my good friends in the customer ranks who may want to know, so take it upon yourself as you see fit to pass the word. Wait a day or so once the process starts, as when I get the call I will be in the hospital in less than 2 hours from the call, and a few hours later, they will make the decision to accept the donor's lungs if judged acceptable, and then they start removing mine.

That initial decision is very critical and the surgeon makes it with confidence, or he sends me home to reset the process for the next chance of fate. Sometimes, a patient can go through this process more than once, but because the surgeon needs to be absolutely sure, he has to be sure in his mind. These thoracic surgeon guys are pretty darn good, and I trust their judgment, I guess you might say with my life, as Gus would say—*duh?*

My e-mail address will be set with a message saying I am out of the office on a medical leave of unknown length, and when you see that, I will be in the hospital for 3–4 weeks. If someone wants to get hold of me, suggest they send an e-mail to my e-mail address, and when I start looking at them, I certainly may feel like responding or calling if that is the case.

With any luck I will be back on e-mail a week or so after surgery, and intend to keep active, so keep me copied on what is happening, as I will want/need things to do.

Once I get out of the hospital I will be limited to home for 6–8 weeks and regular visits to the hospital as the doctors keep a close eye on me for the rejection issues associated with transplant. I have read and been counseled a lot, but I will be learning more as I proceed. This is a fascinating process, and I have truly good fortune to be living 45 minutes or less from this medical facility.

I know I can count on each of you to keep our company moving forward during this medical journey of Spring for me. Hopefully after they plant those new lungs in me, I will be out traveling again by fall. I look forward to that.

Best regards,

Jim Uhrig

CHAPTER 7

Judy Murphy

(written by Travis Murphy, her oldest son)

There are those phone calls that everyone has received or will receive someday. It's that call that comes in the middle of the night, and as soon as you see the number, you know they shouldn't be calling at that time; you know somewhere deep inside that the subsequent conversation after hitting *answer* will change your life. For Jim, it was a call that came in the middle of the night from his doctor on April 20, 2009, telling him that there was a donor match for a set of lungs that he so desperately needed to live. For me, that call came just forty-eight hours earlier from my brother, who opened the conversation simply with, "Something's happened to Mom."

My mother, Judy Annette Snook (Murphy), was born on February 27, 1958, in Topeka, Kansas. Her father spent most of his career as a small-town newspaperman, and her mother occupied herself raising their six kids, my mother the youngest. My mom was also denied the opportunity to see her mother become a grandmother to her children. Her mother, Marie, died while giving birth to her seventh child in 1963. My grandfather remarried soon after, and the woman I always knew as grandma raised my mother from the age of six on.

My mom graduated from high school in Natoma, Kansas, in 1976 and, a few months later, married the boy who had innocently asked her if she wanted a ride home from school when she was a freshman. My dad, Mark Murphy, was the son of a hardworking farm family who had dreams of operating his own large-scale livestock operation. Less than a year later, I came along, and they named me Travis, a name that my dad had always liked. Three other boys—Tyler, Tane, and Tragen—followed me. My mom once told me that she and my dad were going to name me Leslie had I been a girl. It's a good thing I wasn't a girl, as it would have really thrown off the Murphy family naming schematic of all Ts.

My mom was a young nursing student at Butler County Community College, Kansas. She and I would load up in the car every Sunday evening and head to El Dorado from our home in Fredonia, both in southeast Kansas, where my father was managing a small confined feeding hog operation. My dad's work dictated our movements during the early years of our young family and found us moving seven times in my first six years. It seems as though it must have been disruptive, and I'm sure it was stressful in a way that a toddler could not appreciate. Perhaps it is a testament to my parents that I have no unpleasant memories from childhood of repeatedly packing up our things to move to another home, but rather wonderfully warm memories of my mom reading to me and saying prayers before bed: "Now I lay me down to sleep, I pray the Lord my soul to keep." My mom would change the words slightly to take out the reference to dying before I wake in order to protect me, and also her, from what would undoubtedly be a lot of questions.

In 1982, when my mom graduated with her degree as a registered nurse, her family of three looked on proudly, my brother Tyler having been born just a few months earlier. Shortly after, we made the move back to Natoma in northwest Kansas, where my dad had purchased some land to start his own farming operation. My mom found a job at the Russell Regional Hospital, where she would work in various nursing positions for the next sixteen years.

Life in small town Kansas in the 1980s was a sheltered, simple affair. Two more Murphy boys followed: Tane in 1985 and Tragen in 1990. Being close once again to my grandparents, my childhood is marked by holidays—Christmas Eve with my mom's parents and siblings in nearby Hays, Christmas Day at Grandpa and Grandma Murphy's farmhouse. My mom's family had spread out after leaving home, with her siblings moving to Maryland, Hawaii, Arizona, Nebraska, and Missouri. Christmas Eve was always the time that they all came back together, and, as a result, it was my mom's favorite holiday. Over time, when my grandparents passed away and her siblings' own families grew up, Christmas Eve became a bittersweet affair for my mom. She loved all that it represented to her and all the memories she had, but it pained her to be away from her family.

Birthdays were no small affair for my mother. No matter the demands on her schedule—or the tightness of the family budget during the lean years with four kids and a hog market on the decline that sent my father into the red—my mom always made sure each one of us had a party. For me, being born three days before Christmas held the potential of having a childhood cheated, receiving joint Christmas/birthday presents in a way my cousins born in July did not. However, my mom always made sure that I had a birthday party and birthday presents. Going to the Holiday Inn in Hays for a birthday pool party the weekend before Christmas helped to ensure that I was a popular kid each year around the holidays.

As life has a tendency to do for parents, the years passed by, becoming a cycle of school years and summers, repeated until the children's adulthood. My mom did a good job of encouraging our talents and interests, helping us with homework and also being a disciplinarian when needed in a home of four rowdy farm boys. Each of us picked our favorite sport teams, and each Christmas Mom would ensure that we received gifts corresponding with each. My dad was absorbed in his work and emotionally distant, which led all of us to go to our mother for counsel and consolation as well as to share our victories and failures.

She also became a sports fan as each of us blossomed in our own way athletically, and she was fiercely protective of her cubs—perhaps no place more so than on the field of play. No referee was safe from the red-faced woman in the stands, berating them for making the wrong call against one of her own. My mother was always passionate—about music, about her kids, about her interests, and about life. Not all her passions were so heroic, however. She became an avid *Star Trek* fan completely on her own, an interest that none of her offspring really took to despite reruns of *Star Trek: The Next Generation* and *Deep Space Nine* that were a consistent background to our upbringing. There's a great picture of my mom from a trip to the *Star Trek* exhibit at a casino in Las Vegas. She is beaming while posing with a Ferengi. Her only regret, she would later note, was that she wasn't able to meet a Klingon.

As babies turned into teenagers and teenagers into men, my mom was able to focus again on herself and her own career. For many, this stage of life means gardening and reading. However, my mom decided to recapture those years of her youth that passed by so quickly while raising a family. She lost fifty pounds and started walking each evening. She looked into making herself more attractive professionally as well, becoming an early pioneer of online education. She received her bachelor's degree in nursing in 1999 and her master's in 2006. In that time, she also decided to transition from the more lucrative nursing career, in which she had worked for more than two decades, to teaching nursing to others.

In the summer of 2006, my mom and dad; Tragen, who was still living at home as the youngest; my fiancée at the time, Amanda; and I all flew to Arizona for my mom's graduation for her master's degree. In the photos from that day, her radiant smile and the pride of her accomplishment come through just as clearly as they did on the photos of her graduating from nursing school in 1982. Her work to obtain her master's came not as a requirement to the newly obtained position as a nursing instructor but rather was a result of her own drive and determination to better serve the students that sat before her.

I did not see my mom at work in the classroom, but the enthusiasm she had for life was undoubtedly imparted upon those under her tutelage. At her memorial service, a group of students—through tearful laughter—recounted stories of my mother's offbeat sense of humor and her unique teaching tactics. At one point, they held up a plastic magic wand that would light up and make noise—a tactic she employed to get the students' attention or to emphasize a particularly important point.

Emotion was my mother's first reaction. Everything was the funniest, the coolest, the best she had ever seen or heard. If you told her a story you were excited about, she was twice as excited. She loved to laugh and would often do so even before you reached the punch line of your story in anticipation. If you were sad, she would cry with you, and if you were hurt or angry, she would hurt right along with you. She really did care, though; it was never insincere. As teenagers, at times her comical overreactions were embarrassing in a way that made us squirm as impressionable teens.

I remember once at a basketball game my sophomore year of high school, looking up into the stands and mouthing *stop* to the familiar face yelling at the referees. The fact that the same lungs that provided the air to those insults cast out from the bleachers to the men and women in black and white stripes ended up in a man who spent thirty years as a referee would no doubt be the funniest joke of all to her. She loved to laugh.

My favorite memory of my mom is as a child, when she would clean the house on a Saturday morning. She carried around a box of 45s for thirty plus years and she would set up a stack of records to play while she dusted, vacuumed, and did the dishes, singing the entire time. She loved music and she loved to sing. One knew this if they spent more than five minutes in the car with her. She couldn't help but sing. She also loved to dance. Mom and Dad were always among the first and last on the floor at any dance.

She had other passions beyond the crew of the Starship Enterprise. She loved pigs. They were all over the house: flying pigs, talking pigs, stuffed pigs, pictures of pigs. She also loved purple. Her Christmas present the year before she died was a purple bedroom—carpet and paint on the walls.

She also loved the spring. Lilacs and hyacinths were her favorite flowers. So it was fitting that we put her to rest in the spring, in April of 2009. The sun was shining as bright as her smile. She loved the warmth; how could she not, it radiated out from her. The flowers blooming, the trees coming alive—she loved the spring.

My mother collapsed on a Saturday morning while walking into her bedroom to wake up my father. A cerebral hemorrhage snatched her away as quickly as if she'd been standing in front of a speeding train.

Less than a year before her death, we found ourselves in the car, driving back from the untimely death of an uncle, talking about plans after death. My mom, a career medical professional, made her wishes very clear: "If you can, I want to make sure you donate my organs. I'm not going to have any use for them. And don't you dare keep me plugged in." Little did we know that we would have to honor those wishes so soon.

When my brother called that morning to tell me something had happened to mom, I went immediately to the airport and flew back to Kansas from Chicago, where I was living at the time. My other brothers arrived from Ohio and Arizona. Tragen was still at home, and carries the heaviest weight of having helped my dad with CPR until the ambulance came, all a month before his high school graduation. Pacing the hospital halls, waiting for news, the realizations slowly started to sink in. My unborn children would never know their grandmother's laugh, her smile, her effusive emotion. I realized that they would be cheated out of having such a caring, loving, happy soul in their lives. At the same time, my mom was cheated out of the chance to see her grandchildren grow up.

As they say after death, *life goes on*. It's an adage not lacking in truth, but there's so much more. In the days, weeks, and months that followed my mom's passing, we all got on with our lives and coped the best we could, now missing the emotional nucleus of our family.

About a year after her death, I started looking into reaching out to recipients of my mom's organs, or *gifts*. I had seen videos of donor families meeting recipients that brought me to tears and I wondered, *Who was out there, alive today because of a part of my mom?*

Through the Midwestern Transplant Network, the Kansas City-based organization that handled the donations, our family first received a summary of recipients. We were then able to follow up with anonymous letters to those recipients, telling them a bit about my mom, wishing them well, and opening the door for a response. They maintain anonymity until both sides express an interest in learning the identity of the other. I was scared of what I might find out; my worst fear was that none of them had lived and the small amount of justification that we could find in her death, that parts of her would live on in others, was unfounded. What we received instead was the confirmation that she lived on, in a variety of ways, giving life to others.

My mom's liver went to a fifty-two-year-old gentleman from the Midwest who was married with three teenage children. He was able to return to work, and, according to the transplant network, "He enjoys model building, railroad history, movies, and participating in his church."

One of my mom's kidneys went to a fifty-eight-year-old woman from the Midwest. She had been on the waiting list for more than two years when her call came. She sent a very straightforward note that I think my mom would have appreciated. She wrote, "I know nothing about your mother, but she must've been a kind, caring, compassionate, and generous woman. I could make you promises of what I would do to make our world a better place, but we all know promises tend to be broken and time can cause us to forget—but know this, that not one day, not an hour, or a minute will go by without me thinking of what a blessing you have given me."

The other kidney recipient, we learned, had died a few months after the transplant.

Another letter, from a cornea recipient named Anne Marie, was so touching because she explained how my mom's gift had literally allowed her to see more of her family. She had seven children, fourteen grandchildren and five great grandchildren. She had also experienced loss—losing two husbands at thirty-seven and sixty.

They were also able to recover heart valves, tissue, and grafts of bone and its associated connective tissue that went on to help countless others.

The lungs, as you know by reading this book, went to a salesman and frame maker from Pennsylvania, who has taken it upon himself to make the most of the time he has left to help and to serve others. For

this, my family is so very grateful, and I am thankful that we
a partner for life in this effort.

Five years after her death, I still miss my mom. I miss her laughter, I
miss her sense of humor, and I miss the gushing excitement she had
for life. But she lives on. Her memory and the lessons she taught live
on in her children, her friends, students, family and coworkers. Her
organs live on, as well, giving life to others.

At her memorial services, one of her students read the following poem
that accurately captures my mom's life after her death. Just a few
weeks before she passed away, her class had covered a section on
end-of-life and organ donation, and she had found this poem for the
students to consider. By Robert N. Test, it is a beautiful tribute to the
miracle of organ donation and how, like my mom, we can truly live
forever.

The day will come when my body will lie upon a white sheet neatly
tucked under four corners of a mattress located in a hospital busily
occupied with the living and the dying. At a certain moment a
doctor will determine that my brain has ceased to function and
that, for all intents and purposes, my life has ended. When that
happens, do not attempt to instill artificial life into my body by the
use of a machine. And don't call this my deathbed. Let it be called
the bed of life, and let my body be taken from it to help others lead
fuller lives.

Give my sight to the man who has never seen a sunrise, a baby's face
or love in the eyes of a woman.

Give my heart to a person whose own heart has caused nothing but endless days of pain.

Give my blood to the teenager who was pulled from the wreckage of his car, so that he might live to see his grandchildren play.

Give my kidneys to one who depends on a machine to exist from week to week.

Take my bones, every muscle, every fiber and nerve in my body and find a way to make a crippled child walk.

Explore every corner of my brain. Take my cells, if necessary, and let them grow so that, someday a speechless boy will shout at the crack of a bat and a deaf girl will hear the sound of rain against her window.

Burn what is left of me and scatter the ashes to the winds to help the flowers grow.

If you must bury something, let it be my faults, my weaknesses and all prejudice against my fellow man.

Give my sins to the devil.

Give my soul to God.

If, by chance, you wish to remember me, do it with a kind deed or word to someone who needs you.

If you do all I have asked, I will live forever.

CHAPTER 8

Caregivers

This book is dedicated to caregivers. It signifies how important their role is, and, often, how it is more stressful for them than the patient. If you have been a caregiver, you know this. If you will be a caregiver, good luck. Faith will be helpful to get you through, but the best help for you is the support of your friends and family, and the more help you have networking, the better, in most cases.

If somehow you can also do something to keep your mind off the concern for the patient, so much the better. Computers, tablets, and mobile phones may help, up to a point, but they can also be a distraction if they are not part of your normal lifestyle. Have something to keep you occupied and talking to other people are likely the best things you can do. Prayer or meditation can do wonders for all concerned.

If you are a friend of a caregiver, give extra of your time to offer your words and company as you can. It will mean so much to them. In chapter 1, "Great Partners," I talked about Sully's boss, Tom, who really visited Sully a lot when he had his transplants. Tom will tell you he felt he was a bigger help to Claudia, Sully's wife, than he was to Sully.

The hardest chapter for me to write is this one on caregivers. Being heavily sedated in ICU for five of the first six weeks I was in the hospital, I had a general idea what was going on at times. However, many times my recollection of the details were hazy at best, and often full of hallucinations, common with the new drugs administered to transplant recipients. My chief caregiver was Donna, my wife, who had assistance from our family of five children, Sully, and, of course, Dr. Jay Bhama. All had an active role in being my caregivers, but Donna was certainly the quarterback—captain or leader if you prefer.

We live about twenty miles from the hospital, and while the commute is normally forty-five minutes or less, it is much more challenging during rush hour. We operate two small family businesses, about five miles from our house, and while the employees helped keep the businesses on track, Donna was directly involved every day with the businesses, which have adjacent storefronts in a little shopping center.

She did a remarkable job during the whole ordeal, and all the family looked out for her, as well as for me. They all were outstanding!

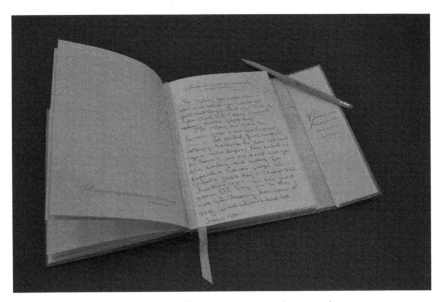

Counting My Blessings, A Gratitude Journal

The family felt it would be a good idea to write a journal about my adventures. The journal is called *Counting My Blessings, A Gratitude Journal*. The entries in the journal were by Donna and my oldest son, Keith. Because of the details they included, it fills in a lot of the unknown issues to me. To help you track these issues, they are included chronologically using some editorial license to help explain, where necessary.

We got the call on April 20, at a little past eleven at night, and I calmly and sanely drove the car and arrived at the hospital about an hour later. While Donna and I traveled together, Robin, Keith, and Ryan met us at the hospital. Kevin and Brad lived in Detroit and were not going to leave Detroit until the surgery started.

The children are from youngest to oldest, Ryan, Brad, Kevin, Keith, and Robin. While I was being prepped for surgery, the others were nervously waiting and learning that the donor was from Kansas and reportedly had died from a stroke. (I learned later it was the result of a cerebral hemorrhage.) A recovery team from UPMC was in route to Kansas.

The donor was, ironically, a nurse committed to organ donorship, and she had died on Saturday, April 18. She was kept on a ventilator while a suitable recipient was found; more details of how I was selected are in chapter 13, "Donors." While her family was suffering agony of such a tragic loss of their mother and wife, my family was wondering if those lungs would work for me to extend my life.

Dr. Bhama introduced himself to my family at around four in the morning, and he told them that he was willing to take a small risk with the donor, which was age-related, but nothing significant. He stated the donor age was the only risk he would accept before proceeding with surgery. He also indicated that the surgeon performing the recovery of the lungs from the donor was very conservative, and would act like he was operating on a member of his family.

The risk factor mentioned is because the donor was over fifty.

Sully showed up around eight in the morning and indicated that since my family was still waiting, that was a good sign, and that the donor lungs appeared to be usable. The doctors arrived thirty minutes later to transport me to surgery.

They started the anesthetic, which they described as tequila-flavored. So I began to sing "Tequila Makes My Clothes Fall Off," a country music song that ironically may make my donor smile, with her fondness for tequila. I do recall singing and hearing laughter in the background from everyone, including the stoic anesthesiologist. Whatever they gave me that was the last I remember until waking up in ICU the next day.

At ten in the morning, Sully indicated the donor lungs would be arriving shortly, at which time Dr. Bhama would inspect them and make a decision to proceed. At 11:07 a.m., the family got the word that the surgery was a go. With that information, my other two sons, Kevin and Brad, headed to the Detroit airport for their trip to Pittsburgh, and also my older brothers, Ron and Bill, made their plans to come.

Now it is about noon; I am in surgery and the family is trying to freshen up and regroup.

With the surgery now underway, the family is trying to relax and is getting encouragement from coworkers at our businesses and those that I work with in my day job. Even some of my customer friends felt compelled to check on me, despite not knowing that I was undergoing surgery that day. I am sure that was uplifting to Donna. By midafternoon, the update report was that one lung was in and working well, while they prepared to insert the second lung. By late afternoon, Kevin and Brad arrived from Detroit to join the family. Around six in the evening a nurse updated the family, reporting that I was doing well on a bypass machine and that surgery should be done in about an hour and a half. A little before seven, Sully had joined the family and was awaiting the opportunity to talk to the surgeon, Dr. Bhama.

Dr. Bhama arrived shortly thereafter and reported that the surgery went well. He was pleased with the process and remarked that I came through the surgery quite well. Two areas of concern were the "freezer burn," attributed to the long commute from Kansas, and how the fragile lungs must be packed in ice, as well as the size of the lungs.

When the cold lungs are introduced to the recipient, the warm tissue and blood can be a shock to the donor organs, causing them to be slow to respond. As a result, my oxygenation levels were lower than he had hoped, and in the mid-90s rather than in the high 90s.

The other issue was that the donor lungs were a bit big for the cavity left by my old lungs, which had shrunk and hardened like two bricks. He said swelling is not uncommon for donor lungs, and they use medication to help address this and to eliminate some excessive fluids that can build up. Accordingly, the incisions for the new organs were not closed. If the shrinkage did not occur, they may need to trim a donated organ so they can close my chest incisions completely. Dr. Bhama indicated this also is not uncommon.

He also commented that the availability of the donor's lungs was fortuitous, as my old lungs would not have lasted much longer. He later defined that—in six to eight weeks my lungs would have failed totally.

By eight that evening, I was on 100 percent oxygenation, and rather than waking me after surgery, they placed me in ICU for the night. But before I was placed there, my family had a chance to visit me and see that I was resting peacefully. Having five children supporting my wife, Donna, and, of course, my successful surgery, was most uplifting to everyone. The calls from outside the family continued.

The next day by late morning, all of the family had visited me and talked to my nurse Jan. Jan related that I had a very good night and was not able to talk, so I wrote notes and drew a family tree of sorts. Being a salesman by trade, I was frustrated by not being able to speak, but I made up for that by writing notes.

Jan, my RN clinician, wrote an entry in the book that the family and I treasure. She claimed I "was an excellent patient and a joy to take care of" and that I was doing great—and asked me to stay in touch with ICU as I am definitely one of the "lucky ones" and "God blessed."

It is ironic that her entry into the journal was adjacent to a quote written by Maltbie D. Babcock that reads: "Better to lose count while naming your blessings than to lose your blessings to counting your troubles." I thought I had that attitude from the start with my diagnosis of pulmonary fibrosis and the possibility of transplant surgery.

I have learned since how lucky—and definitely blessed—I truly am, and only hope my experience can give hope to others facing such a life-changing situation. *Keep the faith* is my signatory I use in many e-mails and book signings always, as that had been instilled in me often with the ups and downs that can occur in anyone's life.

Shortly after noon, Dr. Bhama told the family that I was doing well and the follow-up surgery to close the incisions would be at seven the next morning.

Back to my odyssey—on Wednesday afternoon, the day after my surgery, Donna, my four sons, and Uncle Bill, my brother, all had their own odyssey and went and had a beer "for me." They all sure had earned some relief and, with beer breath, came back late afternoon to find me doing well, and keeping everyone laughing.

By six in the evening, I wrote them all a note to go home and that I loved them, so Keith went to his house, but the other three boys came back to our house for steaks on the grill, and well-deserved relaxation in the hot tub with beers on our deck.

Now it is Thursday, and a little after six in the morning. Donna, Kevin, and my brother Bill are in the room and report that I was quite agitated. I had written a note that read: *I am ready, R U?* As the story goes on, Donna said she was ready but didn't know what for, at which point I flipped the bottom of my gown up causing uproarious laughter.

Reportedly, I seemed a little more confused and confessed to an obsession for banana popsicles. I left for surgery a little before seven to have my incisions closed from the transplant two days earlier. Donna brought my stainless steel cross the day before, and before I went to surgery I gave it to Kevin to hold. All of the family continued their wait during this next surgery, which lasted several hours, and at a little after noon, I was back in my ICU room.

Dr. Bhama visited again to report that they did not have to trim the donor lungs. But the lungs were not working quite up to par since the donated left lung was out of my cavity for almost nine hours before insertion, which is about double the time they hope. Still, he feels I'm doing quite well and is very encouraging to the family.

Meanwhile, in western Kansas, the family and friends of Judy Murphy had gathered to lay her to rest, and her oldest son, Travis, delivered the eulogy, five days after her being declared brain dead. That makes my problems rather insignificant in retrospect, but her wishes to be a donor and donor advocate were honored and filled by her loving family.

One could not be more blessed to have her lungs and spirit as part of one's life.

It's not until you realize that you will not make any more new memories with someone that you really take a look at the memories you have. And you can more fully appreciate how truly grand they were.

In the midst of everything over the last five days I have forced myself to pause and remember things about her. Things that I've always taken for granted or that I found annoying that I would now give anything to see her do again.

She loved to help people. And she did it throughout her life. And now even in death she does the same. She insisted on being an organ donor. So we as her family and friends can take comfort in that she's still giving, still helping, even in death. Right now, there are families who are now able to spend a few more hours, days, weeks, months with one of their loved ones because of her love of helping others.

—Travis Murphy eulogizing his mother, Judy, my donor.

That afternoon I appeared to be in pain, but held everyone's hand, and touched their hearts as an unspoken sign of my love for them. Everyone left for the day, but all were concerned that recovery was a long distant goal. My three younger sons, Kevin, Brad and Ryan, broke the tension later that night by taking aim from the hot tub at the wind chimes on the back deck with empty beer cans. Donna commented that was a great stress reliever for her, and obviously, for my sons.

Donna also received phone calls from my primary care doctor, Dr. Mally, and from George Geyer, a friend who since then also developed IPF and received a lung transplant in October 2013. Ray Flynn and so many other good friends called. Ray later died of esophageal cancer. Unfortunately, there are no transplants for cancer.

All now realize that I was sicker than they ever knew, and even my pug dog, Captain Morgan, seems to be more concerned over my absence.

On Friday, Dr. Bhama indicated I needed more rest, and would stay on the respirator for another day. My x-rays showed some fluid around my lungs, so rest will be the best thing for me. Maybe because of my personality, rest has been difficult.

After lunch, the family reports through Jim (he is from England and a very good nurse) that I'm having hallucinations, which could be caused by the medicine, the lack of sleep, or the combination of both. I finally do fall asleep for three hours or so, which appears to help, and the family goes home around six in the evening.

Early the next morning, the nurse reports I had a restful night, and by midmorning my family reported that I looked much better—yet my breathing tube would remain in place, despite my displeasure with it. My nurse was named Carol, and several of the early nights in ICU, I remember her soothing singing of "Silent Night" that she did for me on request, which gave me peacefulness.

This is now Saturday and all the children and my grandson Tyler are visiting me. My brother Bill is joined by my older brother Ron and his wife, Harriett, all of whom lend their support to me and to my wife and family.

Perhaps, the best partner of all is Sully, who paid a visit at six in the evening and said the *Our Father*, as he is a Eucharistic minister. Donna writes she could not have gotten through this ordeal without Sully, and I am sure she is right. His experience and knowledge is comforting and while he does this support for many patients, he certainly gave Donna special care.

On Sunday the plan is to remove my breathing tube, but a new personal crisis has occurred. The small stainless steel cross that I clutch and rub constantly is missing. Jim, being the dutiful nurse, is looking earnestly for it, and even has alerted the hospital laundry to be on the lookout.

After asking the family to leave, Jim proceeded to give me a bath in the bed, and in doing so found my cross.

Quite appropriately, my cross was sticking to my butt, or in other words, "My ass was on the cross," which certainly provided more than enough encouragement for my sons to practice their aim at the wind chimes while they emptied beer cans for another night in a hot tub.

It was quite a day and even Jim, the nurse, stayed over so he could hear my voice after the breathing tube was removed. My first request was for banana popsicles and Vernors Ginger Ale.

Now it is Monday and the seventh day after my transplant, and I sampled some popsicles and also some ginger ale, but unfortunately the popsicles needed to be sugar free. Dr. Bhama was quite upset that I had anything before I completed the swallow test. The swallow test basically convinces the doctor that no liquids are getting into the lungs when they are swallowed, as this could be very damaging to the transplanted lungs.

Ironically, one of the nurses, Kim, was involved in the popsicle episode and guilty by association. I guess Dr. Bhama forgave her, as they were married two years later! I refer to this as the "Popsicle Police" event and perhaps love blossomed at my bedside.

Eight days after my transplant, I got out of ICU and went to the transition floor, so I was making pretty good progress and a clear liquid diet was on my menu. My oldest son Keith stayed with me the evening I was transferred to my new room, which was quite an adjustment from the intensive care nursing I had up to that point. In ICU, the care is pretty much focused from one nurse. On the transition floor, your nurse will have more patients. The other issue on the transition floor is the noise level is much higher.

As Sully will later relate, I was not nominated for any "Patient of The Year" awards and caused many nurses more grief than any other patient. So evidently there was a failure to communicate somewhere.

Regardless, progress was being made. I was doing some walking, sitting in a chair, and getting solid food. My hallucinations continued, and the noise level from all of the monitors needed for me and the other patients was unsettling to me. It was difficult to sleep, as my room was adjacent to the helicopter pad, and most nights there were at least fifty landings to serve several hospitals in the immediate area. I cross-hatched the landings on a piece of paper, as a way to keep score and to confirm the count!

All this added to my lack of sleep, along with the new medicines, which resulted in me staying in a confused state. It seemed like the nights were the toughest for me, and that is when I complained the most to the nursing staff.

On Friday, it was May 1 and our thirty-third wedding anniversary, which was acknowledged on the white board in my room by the nurse's aide. My wife, Donna, spent the whole day with me, despite my somewhat grumpy nature that day.

Ironically, my granddaughter, Bethany, started calling me Grumpy, in about 2000 when she was three or four, and when I asked her why she called me Grumpy, she responded matter-of-factly, "Because you are!" Somehow I will always think her grandmother put her up to that comment.

On this day I made my longest walk, from the room up to the nurses' station and back, which encouraged me and everyone that in another week or so, I may be released from the hospital. My son Brad got me an anniversary card that I could give to Donna, which was a big surprise for her and a memorable anniversary for us.

The get well cards seem to be coming to me faster than Christmas cards. Many are from people I did not realize even knew I was sick. But the word spread quickly, and all were sharing hope and prayers for my recovery. I even was back on e-mail with my laptop. All helped keep the communication going and encouraged me to keep getting better.

The next day was Saturday and the first Saturday in May, which is always the day of the Kentucky Derby in Louisville, KY. Donna is from Louisville, and we had introduced many friends to a great Louisville tradition known as a Derby Party. While we did not have mint juleps in the hospital, my children were present to watch the race, won by Mine That Bird.

I must admit the TV was kind of fuzzy to me most of the time, other than when I watched the Caring Channel, which is soft music and beautiful photographed scenes of nature. Watching this channel and rubbing my cross gave me comfort. That was a good, relaxing feeling for me, as Monday brought some disturbing news for my recovery.

On Monday, the concern was on my white blood cell count. Donna writes I was not myself, and sensed the doctors were alarmed because my white count was triple what would be normal. I had no fever, but I seemed more confused.

The next day, my white count was double what it was the day before, which is extremely high and necessitated calling in the infectious disease doctors. By Wednesday, my white count was down slightly, but still Dr. Bhama indicated surgery was needed to clean the space around the lungs.

Fourteen days after the second part of my transplant surgery, I was transferred back to the operating room to try to remove the infection from around my lungs. The surgery lasted for five hours and went well, but I was returned to ICU late that evening for what appeared to be starting all over again in ICU. They put me back on the ventilator and inserted a feeding tube, which I shortly thereafter pulled out. I was not a happy camper.

Twenty days after my transplant, I appear very tired and the worry and concern of my family has increased. My temperature is 100 and the doctors are considering placing me back on the ventilator (again). Dr. Bhama says the infection made me weak and very sleepy, but he has confidence I will improve and return home to a full life. He encourages everyone that this is just a little setback.

The next day I was very agitated and complained to the nurse that my wife, Donna, had not been there for two weeks. I was having problems dealing with reality.

I often was asking for ice to cool me off and now needed ice for my sore butt. Lying in bed was not comfortable, and I often preferred to sit in a chair. But I needed pillows to sit on and wanted constantly to go from the chair to the bed, and then back to the chair.

Yes, I was Grumpy—so what?

I pulled out my feeding tube *again*, so I am really a nuisance to a lot of people. Dr. Bhama called Donna to tell her that, despite all of this, I really was getting better, even though his phone call was alarming at first.

Our daughter, Robin, stopped in after her night duty as a nurse at another hospital and helped check my charts, and also helped give me more comfort than the normal duty nurses would be able to offer. Robin's coverage first thing in the day, and then by Donna in the midday and by Keith in the evening—was getting me plenty of comfort and attention.

Being in ICU limits your ability to do much other than rest, and the next day when my wife asked what pain level I was at, I simply gave her the "one" middle finger. Her entry in the book is hopefully that tomorrow will be a better day. No votes from her for the patient of the year either!

The next day was a Friday, and Donna spent most of the day with me, only to learn in the afternoon about a fear that my left lung may collapse. A CT scan revealed I did not have a collapsed left lung, but they did a bedside bronchoscopy, which I did not tolerate very well.

Saturday started better and Keith was on duty first and thought I did well. But by the time Donna arrived in the afternoon, I was going downhill. They put me back on a ventilator and a trach was to follow.

Welcome to Camp Happiness (*not*) again.

Sunday finds me bloated and not doing well—and reported to be very swollen—and Tuesday (four weeks after transplant) the trach was installed. Dr. Bhama did the surgery after being out of town a few days.

This seems to be a turning point in my recovery physically, but mentally I was reported to be depressed, and probably really tired of ICU and particularly of one nurse, who is less than a favorite for most. Donna called her Nurse Ratched and I suspect she may have had good reason to be grouchy, since she had to take care of Grumpy (me).

Because of the trach, I cannot speak unless they have a voice ball included, which mostly is not in, so I am writing again, notes about everything and anything.

Grumpy with pen in hand is not a happy camper.

The next day, ICU *special* nurse Angela came in and told Donna and me that we were going for a date. By the time she had me in a wheelchair and loaded with all of the monitors, it seemed like an hour passed by.

She took us to the garden located on the third floor of the hospital. After all of that effort, when we got there, it was beautiful. I lasted about fifteen minutes before claiming exhaustion and went back to bed. It was a great gesture on her part, and Angela did that for us once again while I was in ICU this second time.

Thursday was the next day and I had a new nurse, Kevin, who everyone liked, and he took me for a walk. Dr. B thinks I am getting a whole lot better. Robin checked me out and approved as well, and Keith and my grandson Koby came in to watch the Pens play in their run for the Stanley Cup.

Despite all this, my temperature spiked to 104 as a result of a kidney infection, and, over the next twenty-four hours, the temp subsided. Heading into Memorial Day weekend, Dr. Bhama said, finally, that I might get back to the transition floor early the next week and then go home a week or two later. *Hooray!*

Nothing gets done over a three-day holiday weekend in hospitals, as no one is working other than just the essential personnel. I remember our daughter Robin and her family and in-laws coming to see me on Monday, which was Memorial Day. We had a nice visit, and for the first time since I got back to ICU, I felt like I was ready to leave and get back to the transition floor.

There are a lot of dedicated nurses and medical personnel to thank after such a long hospital stay. Every year on Good Friday I take the hospital staff a solid chocolate Easter basket full of goodies and a note of my appreciation. I have done this every year since my transplant for ICU, and in the last couple years expanded the basket giving to the nurses on the transition floor, too. While I'm sure they appreciate the chocolate, I also give them a handwritten note expressing my gratitude for their care.

This year (2014) I will give them this book.

The week after Memorial Day, I did make it back to the transition floor, where I stayed for two more weeks prior to being released. The daily entries in the journal end on Memorial Day, which is a good indication that this stressful time I spent in ICU was behind me.

All of my children supported each other and supported Donna, to say nothing of all the great support from our friends and business associates with their phone calls, letters, e-mails, and personal visits made to me and my family. All were such great partners for life, and the networking among the various circles of friends was remarkable.

I had many visitors, and know that my condition many times was not up to the excitement of the company, but the visits were always well appreciated. I have not been back to the hospital other than routine checks in over four years since my transplant. This is rare, and indicative of the great care and surgery I had from the hands of Dr. Bhama and the staff at UPMC. Obviously the care for me was exceptional, but the care the hospital—and especially Dr. Bhama—showed for my wife and family was also exceptional. Sully helped the transition of relationships from his friends in the hospital many times, as he continues to do almost on a daily basis in his volunteer role at UPMC. Sully was always a good friend and coworker and a great mentor as a partner for life for me, Donna, and my family.

CHAPTER 9

Staying Well, After Transplant

One of the biggest challenges after the transplant is to stay healthy and keep active. This sounds like a simple task, but it is often the most challenging and requires great attention to detail. Since your donor made the ultimate sacrifice for your transplant, you should be appreciative of your second chance at life, so listen and learn as much as you can to survive, or—as maybe preferred—*thrive!*

There is no need to be paranoid about risks, but you need to be mindful of them in everything you do, touch, and eat, even to this day. It is important to be cautious about germs, such as things you come in contact with through touch.

Can you say *hand sanitizer?*

Use it, and wash your hands often.

As stated earlier, we need to listen to our medical advisers closely and to other knowledgeable sources. As you read this book, hopefully you find the advice to be a helpful source, but most importantly:

> • This book in no way replaces the professional medical advice by your post-transplant coordinators and doctors.

There will be plenty of risks associated with your staying well and getting stronger after the completion of your transplant. To improve your chances of being a successful transplant recipient, you need to get rest, take your medications, and exercise. Another aspect of getting better is doing something mentally challenging, and if you can combine exercise with that mental aspect, all the better.

While in the hospital, you will rely on the nurses and doctors to see that you get the proper medication and exercise for you to get well enough to go home. When you come home, your caregiver will be important in continuing to see that you get your medications at the proper time. Home nursing options are another potential support network, and yet another option may be extended rehab at a nursing facility before finally getting home.

With a lung transplant, even if you are released to go home, you need to stay reasonably close to the hospital for a few months in case rejection issues occur. Not everyone is from the Pittsburgh area like I was, so a stay at a local residence, or perhaps, the wonderful Family House homes in Pittsburgh could be used.

However, as soon as you are physically and mentally able, you should want to take ownership of taking your medications as prescribed. For me, that was about a month or so after I came home from the hospital, but for others it may be sooner or later—but I would suggest the sooner the better.

This will give you a much better understanding of what medications you are taking, and what their purposes are. In my case, it wasn't until close to six months after my transplant that I understood what the different medications did. More importantly, I immediately learned the need to take the medicine, and timely as it was prescribed.

What if you miss a dosage? Certainly patients can have this happen. It is important to not duplicate or double up your dosages, for you may be possibly confusing your system if you try to do so. The first time you forget your meds, a call to the post-transplant coordinators to report the dilemma will assure you that this happens, but starting with the next dosage, you need to reestablish your set routine of medications.

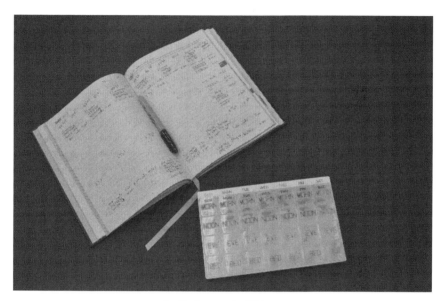

Daily log and pill box

Keep a daily log with all of the medications you take every day. Mine is simplified, as the morning meds and evening meds are defined by prescription. The morning meds are taken at 7:15 a.m. and evening meds 7:15 p.m. If for some reason I feel the need to take Tylenol, or have a new prescription for another issue other than my transplant, I would also enter this in my daily log. An example would be an antibiotic for some unrelated issue, but still logging it in your book is the best advice.

Take that daily log with you to the follow-up doctor visits, for over time your meds will change based on blood work. As the prescriptions change, it is really important to note how your vitals are impacted, or just how you feel, as some can impact your balance or cause swelling. Make notes about that in your log, so you can discuss the specifics with your doctor.

Start out each day with a daily log entry of your oxygen level and pulse rate from a pulse oximeter, your temperature, and your blood pressure. After doing this for several years, you will know when something is a little unusual, like temperature or blood pressure. For example, I know that I have missed my morning meds or evening meds only a few times since my transplant five years ago.

You can use your cell phone as an alarm system, which is a reminder to take your pills. Donna suggested this system, and it has worked very well, but sometimes you may get distracted by a phone call or activity. When you know you are going out to dinner or an evening event could be distracting, take the evening meds an hour early, as the goal is an eleven- to thirteen-hour window. Most meds missed for me were the afternoon ones, and there are just fewer distractions and perhaps more routine in the morning, but establish a routine you can manage best for you.

Whatever system you develop, you need to take ownership of the responsibility to take your meds. You can get in tune with this concept even while still in the hospital; I used to remind my nurses if my evening or morning meds were not administered in the two-hour targeted window for them. I found this endeared me to the nurses looking after me and probably explains, again, why I did not get any votes—let alone nominations—for the coveted "Patient of the Year" award. In reality, the nurses get busy too—which is understandable— but when I was feeling the worst, they were always tracking my meds closely.

For the exercise part of getting better, a physical therapist will start you walking in the hospital. If you have stairs to climb, they will work that into your workout as well. While the hospital has physical therapists who work with you, they are only trying to get you physically strong enough to go home. Once home, it is important to be evaluated by home health-care nurses supplied from your hospital or insurance group.

You will next start physical therapy, which should be done with nurses and physical therapists to monitor your oxygen needs and increase your strength and balance. Simple walking and any other motor skills exercises are good to perform on a regular basis.

One of my goals was to get back on the golf course, so I started putting a golf ball in my living room and then tried to swing a golf club outside. Six months after my transplant, in November 2009, I played nine holes of golf with my grandson and oldest son.

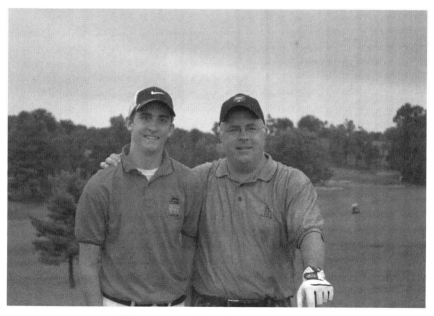

Oldest son, Keith, and grandson Koby

I set this goal when I was in ICU, and they visited me often. We used a golf cart, but my score for nine holes was similar to what I normally shot; I could not go any more holes, as the nine holes were the limit my strength and stamina would allow. In the spring, I started playing more and played in the 2010 Transplant Games in Madison, Wisconsin, fifteen months after my transplant (July 2010).

This was not an easy task, as I built my strength up gradually to eventually be able to play every day, two weeks before the games. While I played golf in the 2012 Transplant Games in Grand Rapids, Michigan, I also ran the one-hundred-meter dash. It was not a matter of running fast, but rather being able to run the race as fast as I could and complete it.

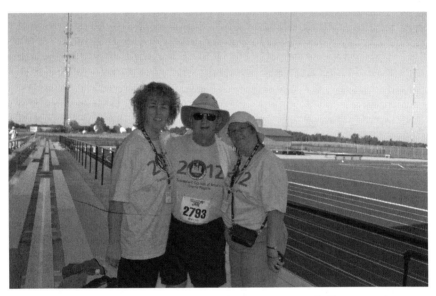

Cardiothoracic Transplant Coordinator Nurses Shelley Zomak
and Colleen Yost with me at the 2012 US Transplant Games

Even to this day, I feel my physical strength is getting better, and in 2013 I was hopeful to go to the World Transplant Games in South Africa in July. My doctors and medical community endorsed my efforts, and I thought of it as another gratifying way to thank my donor. However, after careful thought I decided to not attend those games, as the long flight and crowded airports and planes did not seem to me or my wife to be the best place for a lung transplant recipient. The concern of the time it would take to travel back to UPMC was also an issue, in case I took ill. While other hospitals are always an option, I would feel more confident in returning to UPMC with their direct involvement with my transplant.

On the mental side, because of my extended stay in ICU, and two full months for my hospital stay, my brain functions had been slowed greatly. While able to read e-mails, cards, and documents, it was initially hard to comprehend technical concepts or complicated conversations. About two months later—perhaps as I was becoming more accustomed to the drugs or maybe a slower style of thinking—I went back to work in my day job, five months after my transplant.

My job was as a sales and marketing manager, so the daily routine involved looking after orders and details of orders for our customers and the salesmen who worked with me. Traveling was limited mostly to one or two nights on the road before coming back home from any business trip, breaking back into my old work routine gradually.

As a sales manager, I had a lot of customers to visit, and while most of the travel was by car, occasionally I would have to fly somewhere. If you travel, carry a surgical mask that you can wear when flying, or in a high-risk situation that could be germ laden or dusty. For example, when cutting grass, if the grass is dry or leaves are present, always wear a mask because of the risk of fungus—like *aspergillus*. If the grass is wet, and hence there is no dust, maybe you will not wear the mask. Managing risks is key to success, so be smart about it.

In addition to having my day job, I own a custom picture frame shop with my wife. In that business, our customers bring art, photographs, or perhaps memorabilia to be placed in a custom frame. Our shop is complete, in that we cut the frames, mats, and glass and assemble the frames—all on our premises. While we have employees to help in aspects of our business, I would also do the framing on the weekends and in the evenings, as my day job schedule would permit.

Making a picture frame is task oriented. That is, to make a frame—perhaps like baking a cake—you start with a plan, and when the project is done, it is something people can see visually and appreciate or enjoy. This gives you self-satisfaction and also a sense of accomplishment, which is important in your recovery, especially with drugs that can slow your thought processes down.

There are many transplant recipients who have not gone back to work or become active in any type of activity. Some have become rather sedentary or perhaps medically never recovered or adjusted to the meds. A primary reason I am doing well after nearly five years since my transplant is that my activity level is high, but frequent rest times are still needed. At the end of the day, it's important to rest.

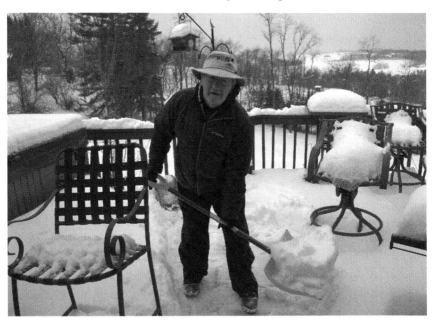

Enjoying shoveling snow again

While your transplant doctors and support personnel are important, you also need to make a visit to the dermatologist or *dermie*. Because of the antirejection drugs or immune suppressant drugs we take, any natural resistance to skin cancer will now also be challenged.

Even before your transplant, you need to visit and establish contact with a dermatologist, since the transplant team needs to know if you have any cancer issues affecting your skin. After your transplant, it is important to stay in touch with your dermatologist; I go every six months. Ironically, on my visit in the fall of 2012, I had a small mark on my nose that the dermatologist identified as being squamous cell carcinoma. It was removed a few weeks later, and I will return to see the dermatologist every six months, to ensure there are no other issues.

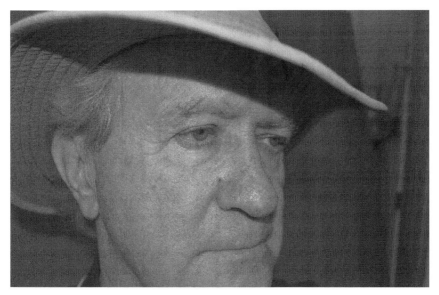

Picture of a developing small squamous cell carcinoma

As for other maintenance issues, any transplant patient—or for that matter *anyone*—should use hand sanitizer, which can be carried in your pocket and car. Wash your hands often throughout the day and especially after touching a menu. I am very cautious about using salt and pepper shakers, and I would never consider using jelly, butter pats, or creamers left on a table in a restaurant. The reason is that with small children handling those items, a virus could easily spread by either touching or using them. Manage your risks smartly.

Go to the dentist for check-ups. I gargle during the day with Listerine; it's a preventive measure for when I feel like I might have been exposed to a cold-bearing person. I did that when I traveled over the years before and since my transplant. It seemed to help prevent me from getting sick and is just good hygiene.

As for a night on the town, take those breath strips in your pocket in case you feel a need for them.

Be very careful and particular about how you greet people. Being in sales, handshakes are common, and in some cases even a hug is warranted. During flu season, you need to be more cautious. It is imperative to get a flu shot every fall, and some transplant recipients get booster shots. Every five years, you should get a pneumonia shot.

These are the things to be mindful of in your daily routine as a patient, so take responsibility to manage this. As a caregiver, you may find yourself being aware of these points as well, but if you want to be a successful transplant patient, you have to assume responsibility to manage your risks.

It is not easy, especially as we age, for things can slow down. But stay determined to put one foot in front of the other every day, and live your life the best you can. Sully instilled that thought in me, and others have reminded me; we owe it to our donors to put forth our best effort. I sure agree with that point of view, now more than ever, since learning more about my donor.

I eventually quit my day job in 2012 to focus on writing this book and also to work full time in the frame shop starting in May of that year. This has also given me more time to be active with CORE (Center for Organ Recovery and Education) and other health-related and volunteer work through UPMC, as you will see in the following chapters.

CHAPTER 10

Bucket List

A bucket list represents the expectations some have for surviving and contains the goals they want to complete. My hopes exceed any bucket list I could create. Perhaps you remember the movie of the same name, with Jack Nicholson and Morgan Freeman, where they both had terminal illnesses and became friends in the hospital. Both developed a bucket list of things they wanted to do before they died.

That may be attractive to some people—and there are certainly some things that one could look forward to doing—but I dare not make a bucket list, for I want to keep living long beyond any checklist is completed. I have a strong feeling to do this for my donor.

A good approach after the transplant is to first listen to the doctors, nurses, and other medical personnel to establish the best course for recovery. As you make progress, you will want to get out of the hospital as fast as you can, but in my case the hospital stay was much longer than average.

After a double lung transplant in 2009, the average hospital time was about three weeks. In my case, after the first week in ICU and the transfer to the transition floor, it looked to everyone that I would be home in the three-week time frame. My physical therapy and attitude were excellent and I was progressing every day.

Unfortunately, after my first long weekend on the transition floor, I developed a staph infection. That put me back in ICU for another month. My second time in ICU was much more difficult than the first week after my transplant. I recall on several occasions having my heart shocked with the paddles to try to settle the heart rhythm to an acceptable rate. If that procedure had not been successful, I may not have survived.

The second time in ICU was very difficult. I was on a lot of painkillers as well as the normal antifungal and antirejection drugs administered normally to a transplant patient. All those drugs combined caused some unusual hallucinations.

While I was in ICU, I started to set some goals for when I got out of the hospital.

My oldest son, Keith, and grandson Koby were regular visitors to me in ICU. In May of 2009, the Pittsburgh Penguins were making a run at the Stanley Cup, and they eventually won it in seven games against Detroit. I think Koby was born wearing skates, as hockey has always been his favorite sport. So it was natural for them to want to watch the games yet also help care for Grumpy, which is the name my wife and granddaughter, Bethany, blessed me with when she was a little girl.

My son and grandson closely watched the hockey games, but in honesty—because of the drugs—I had a very difficult time following the games. As is common with hockey players, many are good golfers, and Koby also loves golf. While we were watching TV and talking, I made a promise to them both that we would play golf in the fall. That was a challenging goal to meet, but in September I was able to swing my driver at one golf ball at a benefit golf outing—but I had no more energy or balance to do more than that, five months after transplant.

By the first weekend of November, my son, grandson, and I played nine holes of golf—not only was I able to do so, but I also beat my grandson by one stroke. Perhaps my competitive nature came out on the final green when my grandson had a six-foot putt to tie me for the nine holes. In true gamesmanship, I asked Koby if he wanted help with reading the putt, and with youthful exuberance he declined and promptly missed the putt to the right. I am considered a very good putter and made putts from all over that ninth green, but with all the drugs I took then, I am probably the last one you should ask to read the line on your putt. Just like most sports, gamesmanship is a part of the game, and perhaps Koby learned a lesson. We all thought back to those Penguins games when I was in ICU and not able to stand up, let alone hit a golf ball.

The second goal I remember from ICU was with my thirtysomething son, Brad. Brad is the next to the youngest of our five children and a big Pittsburgh Steelers and Minnesota Vikings fan. In late October 2009, the Vikings were coming to play the Steelers on my birthday. I had no idea whether I would ever be able to go to a Steelers game again, but I set a goal to do that with Brad. We went to the game, and I stayed for its entirety, watching an exciting Steelers defense score two touchdowns in the final four minutes to beat the Vikings and Brett Favre.

Other than these two goals, I had very little idea of making a list of things I wanted to do—a so-called bucket list. I thought I owed more to my donor. Five months after my transplant, I went back to work as an industrial sales manager and with the related traveling. I may have had a very strange goal for a double lung transplant recipient in his midsixties, but I did want to go back to work, as I felt it would make me healthy and challenge me with a basic regimen each day.

Many lung transplant recipients choose not to go back to work, or in some cases they never get well enough to consider that. Physically and mentally, it is important to make the best recovery you can and to work, if work is an option. If work is not an option, volunteering can be very rewarding, as many of my transplant friends have found.

My travels took me to many places other people may have put on such a bucket list, but I was living my life, doing my job, and trying to get stronger. As I traveled, I met with many partners from the past, some of whom were a big part of my recovery. So, in a way, seeing many of those people were goals, and a very important goal of mine was to thank them and show them my immense gratitude for their support and encouragement.

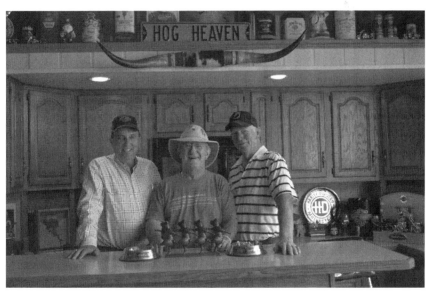

Refractory contractor friends Jim and Joe, prepping
me for the 2012 US Transplant Games.

Since I was in the same industry for forty-five years, most of my customers were family-owned refractory contracting companies, so knowing two, three, and even four generations of people in an organization was not uncommon. Many of the customers and the salesmen who worked with me had very close relationships with me in my career. So it was natural for them to take an interest in my recovery and a delight to see me back to work and getting stronger.

My travels after my transplant took me to New England to visit one of those family companies on a regular basis, and that afforded me the opportunity to visit many landmarks and historical places. By driving and trying to avoid cramped airplanes, that would decrease the possibility of infection from surfaces and in the recirculated air. This resulted in many long drives at my own pace in the eastern United States, which helped better control the risks of travel.

Florida was a trip I made several times a year, so many of those locations could perhaps be on a supposed bucket list, but they were actually part of my travel routine. I have now retired from that industrial sales job, and I think in the future I will do some more traveling, mostly by car to see what is over the horizon. This will also help me to thank and pay homage to my partners, spend some time with them, and visit other potential patients for transplant.

Some incredible things may just happen. For example, my company had supplied some products to NASA for their launch pads, so we were the guests of NASA at Cape Kennedy. I saw the final launch of *Discovery*, and shortly after liftoff, we were able to go down on the launch pad, where things were being soaked with water because of the intense heat of the rocket engines. Now that is something no one would likely put on their bucket list, but it came up on the horizon, and I did it and then shared the experience with friends and family.

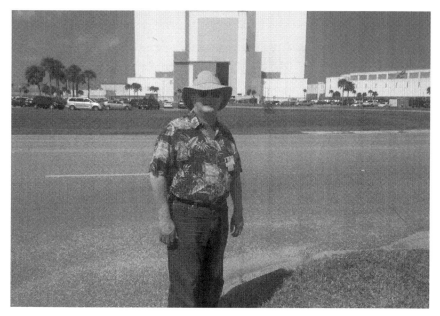

Standing in front of NASA Building in 2012 prior
to the final launch of Discovery.

I guess if there were one thing to include on your bucket list, it would be to make a point of seeing the people who are important to you—especially the partners who gave you encouragement and showed interest in your recovery. They are the best kind of partners, and if you ever get the chance to repay them with a visit, then that will really come easy to you.

Again, I do not have anything against bucket lists, but in my case I'm so busy enjoying and living my second chance at life that I have no plans to make such a list. However, *Partners 4 Life* is about sharing the experience of living a healthy and productive journey. Whether you are a recipient or a partner for a recipient, I hope that you enjoy the journey.

"No limits to what you can do" is a beautiful quote my current pulmonologist, Dr. Morrell, told me after my transplant, but it took me a few years to get there. In the last year I have been cross-country skiing, kayaking, and dancing at my fiftieth high school reunion, and I continue working mostly every day in the frame shop.

Oh, and I was writing a book!

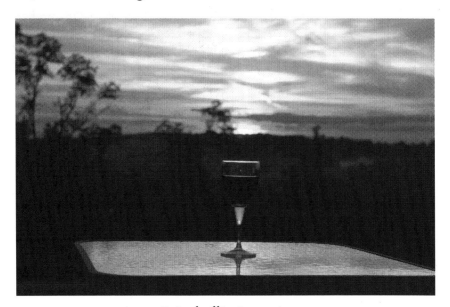

Enjoy brilliant sunsets

More impressively, I know of two women who had double lung transplants; one plays the bagpipes, and the other sings jazz. You may do just about anything if you set your mind positively and have the basic skills.

While enjoying the journey, be ever mindful to give thanks, every day, for the generous gift of life from your donor—and for the medical professionals who accomplish this miracle. If you want to see a gathering of miraculous people, the best place I can think of is the Transplant Games.

These Olympics-style competitions are held in the even years in the United States and in the odd years somewhere in the world, such as in

2013 in South Africa and 2015 planned for Argentina. Every recipient participating recognizes the sacrifices of the donor and their families for their second chance at life. It is a joyful yet very humbling situation that I never thought about until I became a recipient and started walking the transition floors in my recovery. At UPMC, the halls are loaded with pictures from the transplant games and donor quilts where each square signifies a donor story.

Each story is a tribute to the donor; it is heartbreaking for the donor's family, yet a blessing to the recipient. I hope if you are waiting for a transplant, you get the opportunity to have the experience of a second chance at life, which far exceeds any bucket list by anyone, as no one likely has that on their list.

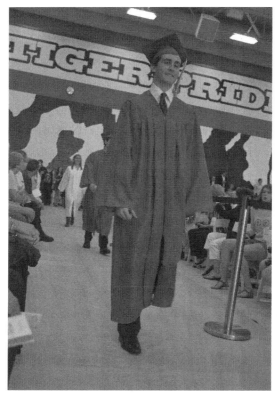

Grandson Koby at his 2013 high school graduation

CHAPTER 11

Helping Others, After Transplant

When faced with recovery after a transplant, your main focus should be on getting better. I emphasized how important going back to some type of activity is for your well-being. In my case, I went back to work as an industrial sales manager, calling on customers and working with my coworkers.

One of my first sales visits was to the buyer of my products for a large company, as my objective was to have a new potential customer. I had made several visits to various people in their plant, to get background and facts before making a proposal to the buyer. Like me, he was a very experienced buyer; as we say, this was not his first rodeo!

I gave him my background and let him know why he had not seen me for several months. Since he was a rather religious person, he was very interested and in wonder of God's hand in these types of things, which I certainly talk about often as well. We had a very good exchange on a personal and business level, and I asked for a trial order, to which he commented, "You are here for a reason and God has something in mind for you, but it is not the product you are trying to sell me."

I did not realize it at the time, but I think the message was clear that my industrial sales job had served a good purpose in my life. But, it was just a vehicle to help me get through life comfortably, help support a wife and five children, and provide for them. I worked hard and was often accused of being a workaholic, but I always insisted my time was not spent just on the work; my passionate focus was servicing the customer, exceeding their expectations, and helping address their needs better than any other supplier.

Some customers welcome that and recognize the experience, product value, or perhaps service a new vendor offers, but in other cases, they may not want to change the pattern of their current thinking and supply. You are not going to be successful in the selling field just because the customer says no; you may need to rephrase the question perhaps, or give up on that business and move on to the next opportunity. It's tough to do that with fewer customers in industry today and more pressure on the salesperson to get business, so this can lead to a different approach.

When it comes to being a new potential transplant patient, it could be similar; getting the best advice is crucial to the patient and caregiver. Doctors and medical personnel can help, and in my case, I had a lifelong trusted friend in Sully who had been down this road not once, but twice for lungs and also once for a kidney transplant.

With Sully as my resource, he got me headed in the right direction, connecting me with the most knowledgeable medical partners specifically for interstitial lung disease. These were the professionals at the Simmons Center whom I refer to in other chapters. Little did I realize how helpful Sully would be to me and my family to get me through the eleven months ahead, after my initial diagnosis in May 2008.

Recalling all of that gives me purpose to help others in other ways.

The first is with the Simmons Center Support Group. This group is run by patients who have been diagnosed with an interstitial lung disease such as pulmonary fibrosis. Dr. Kathy Lindell, PhD, RN, is the main contact from Simmons for the meetings, and the dialogue comes from different speakers following developments in the treatment of the disease.

Since Simmons is a medical and research center and part of a teaching hospital at UPMC, there are many knowledgeable people on the leading edge of finding a cure and researching different treatment options. Some patients have been part of this group since the early days and they have never deteriorated enough to need a transplant. Some have been a member a short time, like me, as I got sicker quickly and Simmons helped me realize that best.

It is similar to having a car problem. Are you going to a regular gas service station or a dealer for service especially for your car type? I go to both, because I know some are really good at certain types of work and others do not specialize. Simmons specializes in this type of disease and I felt immediately at ease with their input and the reality of my worsening condition. I feel that if I did not get their advice when I did, I may not have had the same positive outcome.

This is not the same for everyone. For example, my wife, Donna, did not like to participate in the support meetings, as perhaps she thought it was too harsh a realization of my demise. I wanted to know more and perhaps she might not want to know how bad it was, or at least that was my perception of her lack of interest in these meetings. Even to this day, I try to attend as many as I can to stay abreast of the developments in the research of this disease, as it could one day impact my offspring. I have had quite a few people come into my life—through business or socially—who I have suggested to contact Simmons. It has helped some but not others who were already too far in their progression from this devastating disease.

As I mentioned before another organization I support and proudly work with is CORE, which is the Center for Organ Recovery and Education based here in the Pittsburgh area. Their focus is organ donor awareness and communicating with local hospitals and emergency centers about organ availability. They have recently added in-house capabilities to recover organs at their base facility, and they do so many great things for stimulating interest in organ donation. I have written a chapter about their efforts in this book, and I am one of a number of volunteers who are proud to help CORE.

Family House is an organization that offers affordable housing in the hospital area in Pittsburgh for transplant patients and their families, before and after their transplants. They are a series of big old homes in that section of town similar to large bed and breakfasts, and people come from all over to stay there while they await treatment or observation. For example, after a lung transplant and release from the hospital, you may be required to stay within a certain distance of the hospital for follow-up and closer monitoring.

Often, transplant recipients come to Family House and meet with the patients and caregivers to try to answer their questions and concerns from a fellow patient perspective, like me. Pittsburgh has a high percentage of lung transplants, so there is always someone waiting or recovering who just may want to talk. Sometimes it is only the caregiver, as the patient may be in the hospital.

Here is an example of the gratitude offered and why I enjoy attending these sessions at Family House:

Hi Jo Anne,

Just wanted to let you know (as I'm sure you already do) how helpful the Tx (transplant) support group is for many guests. I just spoke to George Coffey's wife, Tena, from room 56 (waiting for a single lung). She said she had basically given up before going to the support group because all she heard were bad experiences from other Tx guests. She was worried they wouldn't be allowed to have dogs and that her husband George, who is a workaholic, would no longer be able to live an active life. The evening before the support group, she left a disheartening discussion to go to her to room and she prayed to God to hear some success stories. She said the Tx support group was her answer. She was relieved to hear that Jim (Uhrig) leads such an active life (play golf) and that he has a dog! She said, "He gave me comfort that no one else could give me up until that point."

It was touching for me to hear her story and I thought you may want to pass these words on to Jim, and know that your group makes all the difference in many lives! Thanks for all you do, Jo Anne.

Not always do we get a thank you note or acknowledgement, but I welcome the opportunity to help others and give them any comfort I can.

Some of the activities I have done for pulmonary fibrosis awareness and related issues are as follows:

- participated in an October 2009 webinar telling my story
- testified to the FDA on a drug study for Pirfenidon in the spring of 2010
- made a video in 2013 to be used by CORE for primary care doctors and others to show a transplant success story
- local television shows highlighting transplant patients perspectives

- most recently, spoke at an IPF awareness meeting in Harrisburg, in October 2013
- speaking at Rotary, CORE and other interested community and medical groups

Being neither camera shy nor speaker shy, I am willing to talk about the benefits I have had with my transplant to help inspire others to realize the opportunities available. Having given many speeches in my sales career and trained many speakers or helped them develop their story, I am well suited—and blessed—to be able to tell this most important story and hopefully, in return, to help some people, as I was helped.

CHAPTER 12

CORE

I have mentioned the organ procurement organization called CORE, the Center for Organ Recovery and Education. They are one of fifty-eight federally designated organ procurement organizations (OPOs) in the United States. CORE is located in Pittsburgh and close to the action of the major transplant hospitals in the area. They are a nonprofit organization dedicated to promoting donation, education, and research for the purpose of saving and improving the quality of life through organ, tissue, and cornea transplantation.

During my forty-five-year business career in sales and management, I evaluated the performance of companies that did work for my company, as well as companies to which we sold our services. This gave a broad scope and perspective of the efficiencies of business operations. Honestly, CORE is one of the best organizations I have interacted with in business. They have approximately one hundred employees focused on improving the donation of organs, tissue, and corneas—and the most efficient use of those donations.

My volunteer work for them is primarily as a speaker or in an event PR staff function throughout western Pennsylvania and the surrounding area. It has been said that nothing will lighten your heart like lifting the heart of another, which is the essence of volunteer work. It also has been said that the happiest people are those who help others, and

I can attest to the feeling of contribution when I volunteer for CORE and other transplant and donation causes.

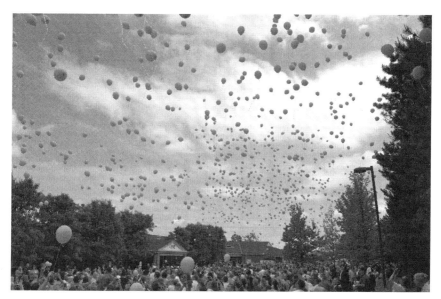

CORE's Annual Special Place gathering, with
families of donors being honored

Many of the personnel at CORE became employees because a loved one was affected as an organ recipient or an organ donor. CORE does so much to comfort the organ donor families, which is an incredibly difficult task.

My first experience seeing CORE at work was with the sudden death of a father in our neighborhood who left behind a widow and two grown children. As the neighbors gathered to offer their condolences at their home that evening, the call from CORE was received, and their sensitivity in a time of intense bereavement for the family was impressive.

I did not connect with the parallel that would occur somewhere if donor lungs came available for me. It was perhaps naïveté or insensitivity on my part, but when you're struggling for oxygen in every breath, you stay very focused just on breathing. But I will never forget that night and the call from CORE to our neighbor friends.

CORE is consistently trying to secure organs and tissues for transplant and improving their methods and capabilities. They are often at odds with coroners and funeral directors, for when a death occurs it may take a couple days—as it did in my case—to match up the available organs with a specific recipient. Some coroners are very responsive to the needs, while others could have a conflict of interest in their ownership positions of funeral homes. CORE works very hard to please all partners in the community of practice, but it is determined to secure and optimize the use of qualified donors.

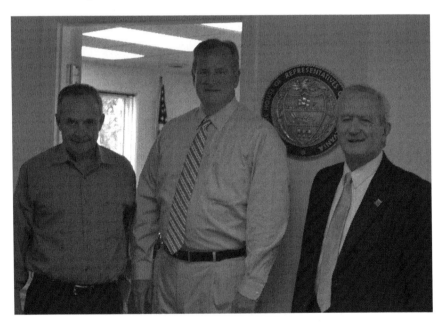

George Geyer and me visiting PA state representative
John Mayer to discuss donate life legislation.

Besides matching the donor with the recipient, often times the delay of recovering the needed organs is because operating rooms are being used for emergencies to save lives, and they might not be available in the timeframe needed. Hospitals also have staffing issues that can add to the delays. The recovery of organs is treated with great respect and dignity, and the medical transplant recovery team assures the surgery is treated as they would if they were operating on their own family member.

To help remedy this specific problem, CORE and some other organ procurement organizations have added their own in-house operating room capabilities. These in-house operating room capabilities are designed to recover the available organs for transfer to the transplant facility and improve recovery time; this could also expedite the funeral process for the bereaved family.

For all transplants, the current statistics in 2013 are overwhelming:

- 120,000 potential candidates need transplants
- 75,000 currently on the active list
- 15,000 transplants done in first three quarters of 2013

We need more donors!

Ask your family and friends to consider making a Pledge for Life by becoming an organ and tissue donor at www.donatelife.pa.com

I have also recently learned that, even as a transplant recipient, you can be an organ donor. I am proud to be one!

CHAPTER 13

Donors

My second chance at life would not exist if it were not for donors, specifically *my* donor, who made the decision to be a donor when asked many years ago. You have read her incredible story in chapter 7, "Judy Murphy," as written by her oldest son, Travis. Not only was she a donor, but also she really taught the importance of donors and organ transplants to nurses, so she was quite the advocate of organ donation.

Perhaps like you, when asked at the driver's license center back in the nineties, I said *yes*, I would be an organ donor. My wife agreed on her license as well and we both thought it was a good idea. It just seemed like the right thing to do, but never did I dream that someday that decision by *another* person would ultimately play the most important part of my double lung transplant—and my second chance at life.

When you are feeling sick and visit the doctor, you try to find out about the condition and the symptoms causing the problem. When I was told I had pulmonary fibrosis, I figured it was just a disruption to my life, but I did not realize it would be life threatening and that over the next eleven months I would be gasping for air. As I learned, this also could impact my heart. The fact that many lung transplants procedures may also include a heart transplant is not a coincidence, as they are closely related.

While some organs (livers and kidneys) can be transplanted from living donors, presently there is no other way to secure a lung or a heart, except by the tragic misfortune of a deceased donor. They are working on other medical options at this time, such as temporary artificial lungs. In my case, I was so sick that I never even thought much about a donor not being available, but obviously that was and is the case for most patients needing a lung transplant.

From a numbers aspect, there are not many lung transplants done annually. In the past year there were about one thousand five hundred done in the United States, and four years ago when I received mine there were only about a thousand.

When you consider PF patients, they number about 150,000 at a given point in time and about 40,000 die each year. The latest stat is that less than 5 percent get a transplant. Those stats can be frightening to someone with this disease, but they are the rough stats; like any stats, they do not tell the whole story, like my story.

I got the best medical advice and support from family, friends, transplant recipients, and support groups. Most significantly, I was matched with a donor who died in the time frame that coincided with my situation. Her sudden demise was due to having a cerebral hemorrhage in her early fifties; she left behind a devastated family of four sons, grandchildren, and a loving husband who had been her high school sweetheart. Countless friends and relatives grieved and missed their vibrant coworker, teacher, or neighbor—or just the smiling, singing, dancing woman named Judy, from Kansas.

She was a very positive upbeat nurse, and very much involved in organ donor awareness and advocacy, according to the letters I received from her oldest son, Travis. There is much to tell about the donor family's side of the story, and his chapter on her life does this.

As a patient with a serious lung issue, I was not focused on organs becoming available, but rather on my constant fear of running out of oxygen. The odds are against you getting a lung transplant. Luck and fate and powers beyond your imagination play a part, but your mental outlook, health, and physical therapy are also important.

I kept occupied by working in my day job up to the day that I was called for my transplant. Perhaps you do not have a job where you can work at home like I did, spending much of my time on the computer or phone. Some people may not be able to work. The biggest benefit of working was that I did not have much idle time to worry about *the call* coming, nor where my donor may come from; Kansas was a long way for Dorothy in the *Wizard of Oz* and Jimmy in Pittsburgh.

So, unbeknownst to me, on Saturday April 18, the fate of my donor became a reality as an organ donor, with her untimely death and the crushing news for her loving family. She lived in Kansas and died suddenly at home, but was kept on life support after being declared brain dead.

Organ procurement organizations (OPO) like CORE get involved at that point to try to find a recipient within five hundred miles of the donor. That area is known as *Zone A,* and if none is found, they move on to one thousand miles of the donor to *Zone B.* (This OPO would have been the Midwestern Transplant Network, the Kansas City-based organization that handled the donations.)

When I got my call I did not know any of that, and over the next couple of months I recall being told that others were offered the organs but had turned them down because they were identified as high risk. High-risk organs are from donors who may have an age issue—such as being over fifty in my donor's case—or uncertain medical history of the donor, as with prison inmates.

The point is that my donor was a nurse very committed to organ donorship, and her family honored her wishes despite the agony of delaying the funeral five days. She died on Saturday, I was called late Monday night, and I willingly agreed to be the recipient of high-risk lungs. A Pittsburgh-based surgical team flew to Kansas City to recover the lungs and bring them back to Pittsburgh. I was transplanted on Tuesday and my benevolent donor was buried on Thursday.

There are so many people committed to making sure donors wishes are fulfilled once that donor commits to be an organ donor. There are fifty-eight federally designated organ procurement organizations (donate life organizations) in the United States, but they are individually operated and in close coordination with United Network for Organ Sharing (UNOS) to match available organs with recipients. UNOS oversees the nation's organ transplant system under a contract with the federal government.

I have come to know a lot more about the OPO in Pittsburgh called CORE (Center for Organ Recovery and Education), where I volunteer. I feel so strongly about their cause and their highly dedicated employees and have dedicated the previous chapter to their efforts. I would not be writing this book without their diligence and excellent work.

I have one favor to ask of you: *if you are not an organ donor, please consider that option.* This can be easily done when you get your driver's license or look on the Internet for www.donatelife-pa.org. In other states, try your state instead of PA or your state's abbreviation. Please just consider it. As a recipient I thought I could not be a donor, but that is not true, and I am a donor—like hopefully you are.

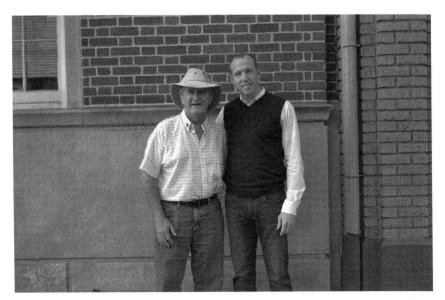

Travis Murphy and I at our first meeting.

I learned more about my donor, as told to me by her oldest son, Travis. Her name is Judy, and I call her *Jude*—as the music she brings me is that of her love for music and particularly the oldies from stacks of 45s she would play doing the household chores on Saturdays. My favorite song in my car is "Hey Jude," and the awesome words of that song bring me closer to knowing Judy and her love of song and dance. Maybe she had a 45 record with this Beatles classic; somehow I think she must have liked it, like I do now.

As a recipient you should consider writing your donor family when you recover, which is a difficult letter to write. Just remember that as tough as it is to write such a letter, it is tougher for the family to respond, and you may not get a response. I wrote mine three months after my transplant when I felt confident to put my gratitude for the gift of life I had gotten in April into words. When I received a letter from Travis addressed to Jim, he started by saying how tough it was to write that letter.

All letters goes through the protocol of being sent to you or to the donor through your transplant coordinator, in my case Shelley Zomak from UPMC. Shelley is the one who gave me the letter from Travis when I was headed to visit a friend, who ironically had just received a double lung transplant himself. It was quite a moment to read his letter and get my initial insight into the life of this amazing woman named Judy. I responded to that letter with gratitude, humility, and assurance to Travis that I would honor his mother's gift for my second chance at life.

Early in 2013, I wrote Travis what I thought would be my final letter. In that letter I told him about my continued good health, improving strength, and my activities in our family frame shop. I also reviewed my involvement with Team Pittsburgh in the US Transplant Games.

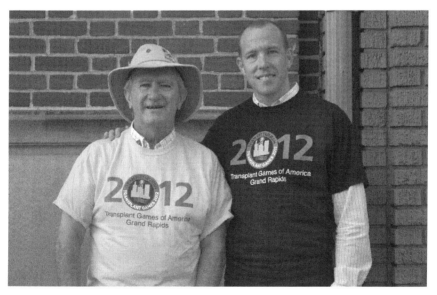

Team Pittsburgh shirts for Travis and me

Those comments about my athletic involvement and volunteer work caught his attention, and his journalist's expertise enabled him to research this guy named Jim from Pennsylvania. Through the US Transplant Games website, he found a runner named Jim on Team

Pittsburgh. He next friended me through Facebook, indicating he was Travis from Kansas and wanted to be my friend.

You can imagine my wonderment and gratitude of such an offer of friendship. I responded that the only Travis I knew from Kansas was Judy's son and that I indeed would welcome the opportunity to be his friend. Since I preferred e-mail, I suggested we resort to that communication method.

Travis has a communications background and works for the US State Department, currently on assignment in Africa. He came to Washington DC for some training updates in the middle of September 2013, and we planned our first face-to-face meeting. He has indicated that he and his family are inspired by my efforts on behalf of organ donorship and other related volunteer activities that I do.

Obviously, with his communications background, he's very interested in a book to help other patients, caregivers, and donors to help honor his mother, Judy. I am so thankful that Travis offered some information about his mother, such as what helped her make the decision to be an organ donor. Another poignant topic is advice he would have for organ donor families to get through the most traumatic event most people could experience—the death of a loved one. His chapter honoring his mother is the highlight of this book project now completed. Yes, I am lucky—but still very blessed.

Like I said in other parts of this book, I would not describe myself as a strongly religious individual, but I did have a great Christian value upbringing and I carry my little steel cross with me everywhere. I pray for a lot of people on my prayer list, and I now have Travis and Jude's family on my list.

Always will.

Author's note:

The actual cross I held during my transplant is no longer with me as I gave mine to Travis when we met in September 2013 with the hopes that it could serve him good fortune, like it did me. I have a few back-ups, but the cross that helped get me through is now serving a new owner, and partner for life, Travis. He gave me his Mother's purple elastic wrist bracelet that says Spirit on one side and on the other, *A Complaint Free World.org*, which I will always wear. Keep the faith.

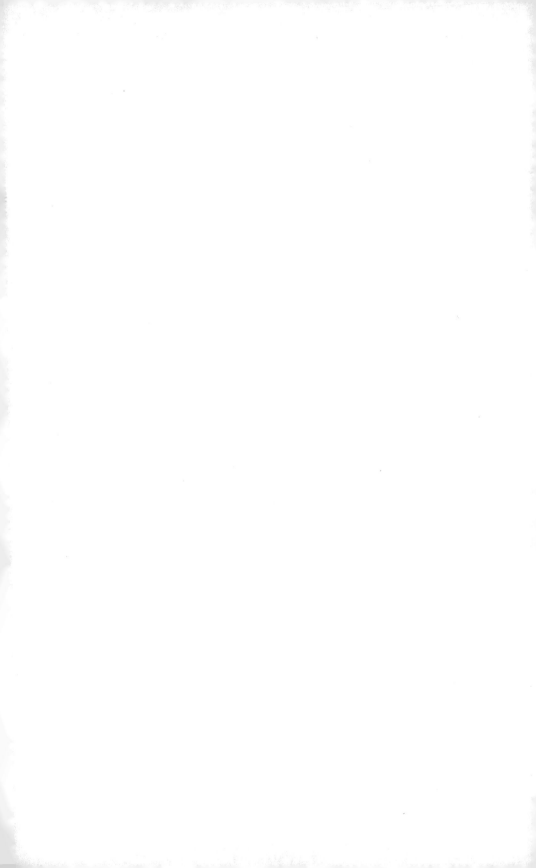

35804045R00083